Y *oga*
O *pening*
U *nfolding*

&

M *eaningful*
E *xperience*

In memory of
my dear friend and personal advisor the late

Beatrice Hope Alexander

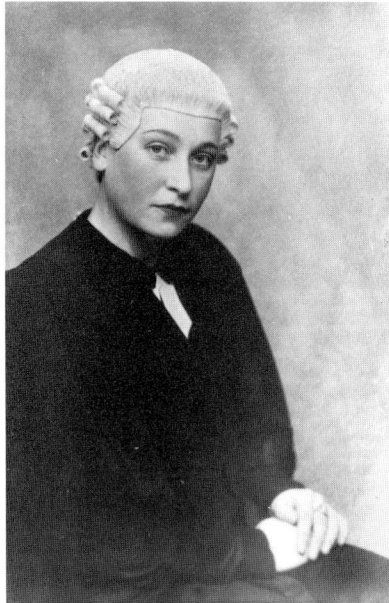

The Origin of the

YOU & ME
Yoga System

Maria Gunstone

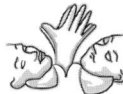

YOU&ME

YOU & ME Publications
www.youandmeyoga.com

Published by YOU & ME Publications
www.youandmeyoga.com

Copyright © Maria Gunstone, 2001

British Library Cataloguing-in-Publication data
A CIP record for this book is available from the British Library

ISBN 1-904117-00-7

Typeset in Century Schoolbook by Carnegie Publishing
Printed and bound in the UK by
Biddles, King's Lynn and Guildford

Contents

Part Three   After India

Part Four   Developing the System

Part Five   Teaching Materials

Foreword

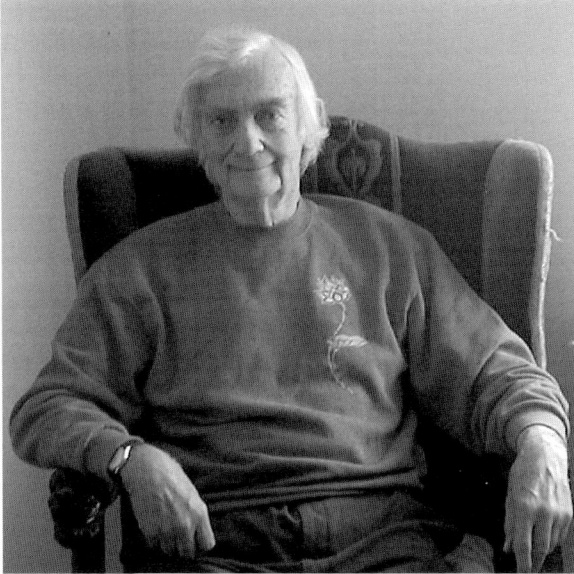

Karma Yoga – the yoga of action – is based on the understanding that we all have a path to follow in this life. How it came about is a matter of great complexity based on the law of Cause and Effect. Because we are so conditioned to make decisions and choices, we are all too often unaware of the action we should be taking, and plough on wondering why life is so unpleasant.

If, however, we do begin to understand what our steps should be and follow that understanding, our lives take on a new dimension. The path is not necessarily easy, but it is totally fulfilling.

Maria Gunstone is clearly motivated by the path which is her own particular karma; bringing new possibilities and hope into the lives of those with a variety of disabilities.

I have known Maria for more than 20 years and have seen, in that time, many of the disappointments and setbacks she has suffered. I have seen her in tears – but I have never seen her lose her sense of determination and dedication.

The knowledge that what she seeks to achieve is what she is called on to achieve, has carried her through many difficult and depressing situations.

Her yoga-based programme is *truly* yoga-based in that it is based on the understanding of union. Maria and her trained trainers share with those they are helping and in no way feel superior to them. While they have specific help to give, they are also always open to receive.

Whatever the problem, mental or physical – almost always both – the 'sufferer' also has a part to play. Something to give as well as receive. This clearly comes through in Maria's attitude.

This story is of a brave woman, who would not be deflected. This text should encourage many more to join her on the path of true union.

Howard Kent
TV Producer, Yoga for Health
Director, Yoga for Health Foundation

Preface and Acknowledgements

When I look back on my early yoga experiences I think I must have had one of the best possible forms of therapy for personal development, despite recovering from a traumatic accident. So I have every reason to believe that miracles can be achieved through yoga!

Nearly three decades on, my YOU & ME Yoga System for people with learning difficulties is the first of its kind to qualify both the students and their trainers. This book includes the development of the system, the teaching materials and the certificated training.

There are five parts to this book: 'My Story', 'India' – an account of my Winston Churchill Fellowship – 'After India', 'Developing the System', and 'Teaching Materials'.

If you hope to visit India to meet the Yoga masters and experience Yoga Ashram life, particularly with a view to understanding the therapeutic value of yoga for different people's needs, this book will be of utmost interest to you.

I am indebted to the late Beatrice Hope Alexander and to Karen Hodge for editing this material, to Ian Douglass and Katerina Kazakina for their proofreading. Also to Pauline Needham for her illustrations. I am grateful to everyone with whom I have had the privilege of working while conducting this mission.

I am thankful to my husband Chris Gunstone who has always been there for me. I am grateful to my mother and family for all their support.

My Yoga teachers (to mention just a few): my first yoga teacher – Jarnine, Sri Paul, Bill Findlater, Ernest Roberts, Malcolm Strutt, Joy Mankoo, Robert Hughes, Howard Kent, plus all the Yoga teachers classes and seminars I attended to obtain and maintain my British Wheel of Yoga diploma.

The Indian yoga masters with whom I had great pleasure in studying: Swami Gitananda, Yogacharya S. Janikraman, Yogacharya B.K.S. Iyengar, Desikachar, Dr M.L. Gharote and Dr M.V. Bhole.

The Winston Churchill Memorial Trust for the travelling fellowship to India, providing me with a magnificent chance of a lifetime. The highlight of my fellowship meeting Dr P. Jeychandran, Director of Special Education in Madras who innovated Yoga in the Special Education curriculum.

My yoga core-group and all the disabled people I have taught yoga and discovered more about the value of yoga. All the trainers and students in the UK and India who allowed me to video and take photographs of their yoga practices which enabled me to produce user-friendly teaching materials.

Valerie and David Tarbuck for their spiritual guidance during the past 25 years. Mencap City Foundation for the grants and support of my work since 1989. The YOU & ME trustees who supported my work. I am particularly grateful for the support and compassion I have constantly received from Jean Millson. The trainers and students in Cumbria who attended the YOU & ME pilot-project. Karen Leslie, Janet Jones, Roger Dangerfield and Jakes Makin who helped make the pilot a success. Charles Tisdall, therapists and staff at Dacrelands Natural Health Centre where I have an office and have received excellent treatments.

The practitioners who have long been waiting for me to publish the training package for them to do the certified training, which motivated me to complete these works.

And last but not least all the students, practitioners, trainers and therapists I have had the privilege in teaching and sharing in yoga.

Terminology used

The term *Trainers* is used for persons qualified to teach YOU & ME to students. The spelling of *trainer* without the capital T denotes those unqualified. The terms *disabled, students or clients* refer to people with learning difficulties and/or disabilities – the current definitions used for people with learning difficulties and/or disabilities. Note that I have used definitions that are in context with the times – throughout the book.

Addresses

The addresses quoted in this book were correct at the time of my Fellowship. I have not had the opportunity to check all of them before going to press.

Part One

My Story

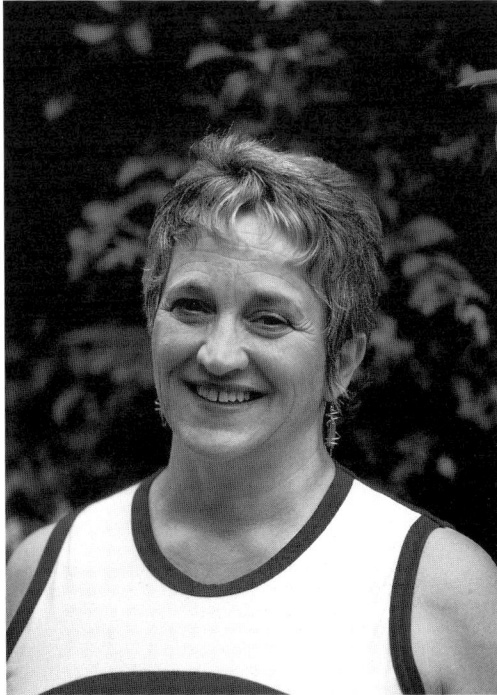

CHAPTER ONE

My Story

In my teens I went to Art College and studied graphics and fashion. Then, in 1972, I suffered multiple injuries in a car accident, which left me feeling that I had lost everything. After 18 days' concussion, I regained consciousness to learn that I had a paralysed ocular motor nerve, a fractured 6th cervical vertebra, and fractured right pelvis. I was confined to a wheelchair and wore a cervical collar for five months. I had double vision and was seeing everything lopsided. Nine months later, I took up yoga and found there was 'light at the end of a dark tunnel'. I saw a way I could improve both my physical strength and my concentration. Having suffered with recurring amnesia for nearly two years after the accident, which was very frightening, I was helped by yoga to regain my confidence. Through the diligent practice of yoga, I made a very good recovery within two years and exceeded medical expectation.

Since 1975, using creative integration group work, I have combined my art training with my knowledge of yoga for disabled people to devise the 'YOU & ME' system. I have produced teaching and educational materials to facilitate practice and motivation to learn.

My Yoga History

I first came in contact with yoga a couple of years before the accident, through the TV series *Yoga for Health* with Richard Hittleman. My mother and I occasionally attempted to follow his instructions and copy Lynne Marshall's supple demonstrations of various yoga postures. Mostly we rolled around the floor laughing, because we had never before attempted to perform unusual movements such as sitting on the floor with the soles of the feet touching and bringing the head down towards the feet. All the while Richard Hittleman drew our attention to think about what we were doing throughout the practices. It was, I suppose, an outlet to laugh at what seemed like 'tying-yourself-in-knots'.

After the car accident, however, I took my yoga practice very seriously. I started with an Iyengar yoga teacher, Jarnine. She was

French and had not started yoga until she was in her sixties, yet she was excellent at demonstrating the postures, and gave her instructions slowly in English. After a year I started attending different yoga teachers' classes throughout south-east London. Within 18 months I was attending a different class twice daily during weekdays and one class on Saturday mornings. In the early seventies most yoga teachers in London were trained in the Iyengar system so I was doing a lot of vigorous physical training and soon became very fit. I gained a lot of confidence and lost the 2 stone in weight I had put on after the car accident.

After three years of intensive practice, during which I gained more mental and physical control and strength, I decided that I wanted to make a career in yoga. I was told by a senior Iyengar teacher that I was not yet ready to teach yoga, and that I should go away and become a nurse, get married and have children – just like she had, in fact – and only then should I consider embarking on such a career.

Yet my heart was set on becoming a qualified yoga teacher, so I set out to find a different route to this end. Fortunately, I discovered a fairly new yoga organisation called *Re-Orientation United Centre Foundation* (ROUCF), a system of classical yoga which opened up a whole new realm of potential and interest.

I enjoyed my training and teaching work and learnt a lot from my teachers, Sri Paul, founder of ROUCF and Bill Findlater, senior ROUCF teacher. Sri Paul, who was originally brought up in a Quaker family, studied yoga in India with Bagwan Maharishi, the well known guru whose teachings are based on the belief 'I AM, THAT I AM', a belief largely to do with the mind and positive thinking. Sri Paul was an expert in relaxation, which was a good balance for me at that time, following my intensive practice of Hatha Yoga during the previous three years. Sri Paul opened the ROUCF headquarters in Notting Hill Gate, West London.

My other ROUCF teacher, Bill Findlater, ran the ROUCF Centre in Croydon, Surrey. Croydon was easier for me to get to, so I attended Bill's students' class and trainers' training, twice a week. He was a qualified school teacher, but found he preferred teaching yoga, which was not permitted in schools for children in those days. Nowadays yoga is reaching many children in the classroom, and is part of the curriculum in some schools – a very good development.

I also attended Sri Paul's monthly meetings for trainers to get together, share our yoga teaching experiences and gain some valuable lessons from Sri Paul. As well as having a good relationship with my teachers, I met some amazing people who also became Yoga Trainers. They were mostly in their mid- to late-twenties, and I think I'm right in saying we all grew together in yoga.

When I look back on all my early yoga experiences, I think I must have had one of the best possible forms of therapy for personal development, despite recovering from a traumatic accident. So I have every reason to believe that miracles can be achieved through yoga! In those days I was an absolute fanatic, which was good because my whole life changed for the better through the practice of yoga.

Grove Park Yoga Centre

I was fortunate to have the use of the upstairs of my father's work premises, an enormous hayloft. He ran a business converting accounting machines to decimalisation. When he heard that I was needing premises to set up a yoga centre for the local community, he offered to move the various pieces of machinery from upstairs down to the ground floor, to give me a big open space for yoga sessions. Soon after, Grove Park Yoga Centre, the third ROUCF centre was established. The space in this hayloft was perfect. In fact there was too much space – being a hayloft there was no ceiling, but a roof of limestone with horses' hair covering, making it difficult to keep in any heat. So, my father fitted plaster boards across the roof beams to form a ceiling. This separated the roof from the stone walls and provided adequate insulation.

Sri Paul offered to officially open the centre, and publicity about this was circulated through the local free newspaper and displayed on the local notice-boards, libraries and community centres. The date was set for three weeks hence. Other Trainers working with me – April, Glenda, Ken and Pete – helped me to decorate by filling in the holes in the stone walls and woodwork. This took a couple of days and involved putting two layers of paint on the walls and ceiling, and scrubbing the greasy floor boards. Once decorated, the original smell of horses returned. The floor was still bare and wood splintery, the windows were bare and the room was too big and open to keep warm. There were six days to opening and we still needed carpets, curtains and heating facilities. In desperation, I rang Sri Paul and asked how on earth was everything going to be ready in time for the opening. He told me not to worry, that he would meditate on everything being ready for the day, and that it would be well attended. He added that I should also meditate for the same good outcome.

Well, miraculously, sufficient carpets and curtains turned up – someone even carried in a carpet they purchased for pennies from a man passing with a rag-and-bone cart! Out of the blue, various friends' family members produced unwanted carpets, rugs, heaters and even a calor gas cooker. My mother found me huge curtains to separate the large room space in two – one end for the practice area, and the other for changing and my office space – and the curtain dividers also helped control room temperature. Sri Paul was more than pleased to see that our meditation had not been in vain and the Opening Day was a tremendous success. The loft area was full with all kinds of people from the local community, mostly people I had never seen before. My peer Trainers accompanied me in demonstrating the yoga practices, while Sri Paul gave explanations of how the ROUCF yoga training programme progresses. A friend took photographs and my grandmother offered to sit in the middle of a circle formed by us Trainers performing Half-Shoulderstand.

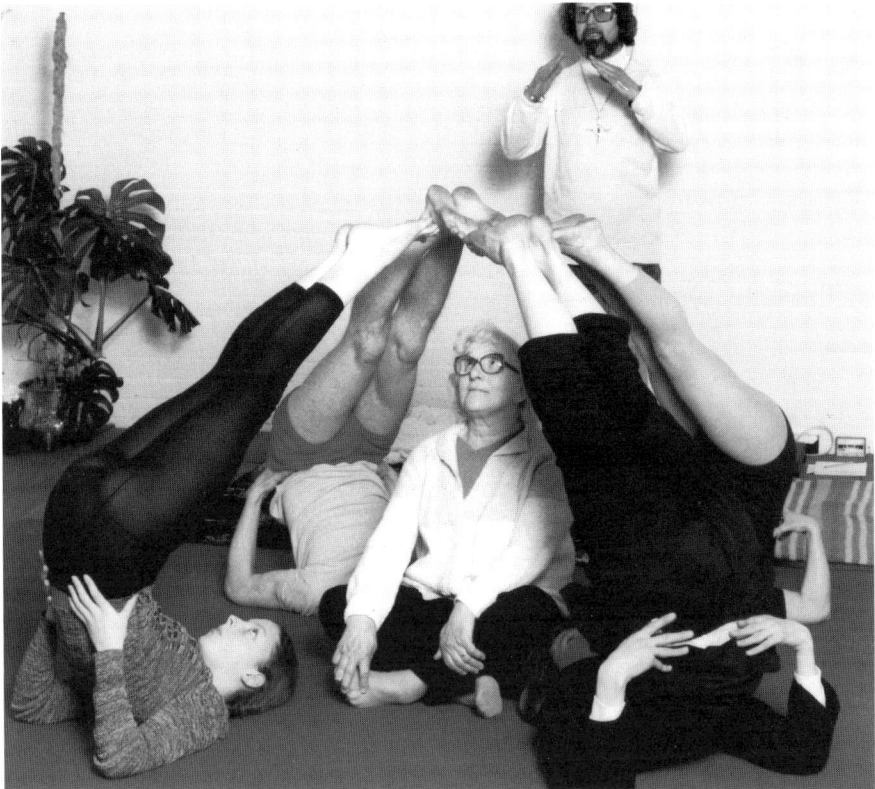

It was a great day. At the end, several people registered for the 12-week Stage One classes due to start on a mutually convenient date. Within six months the centre was fully active. There were morning, afternoon and evening classes five-days a week, with a maximum number of eight students in each class. I employed two registrars to take bookings by making home visits to potential students, and three Stage One students who went on to Level One to become qualified to teach both Stage One and Stage Two courses at the centre.

All in all there were over 500 people who enrolled on at least one of the three Stage courses. It was a fulfilling time for myself and I think the course members had a really good time discovering about themselves and about yoga. Daytime classes were mainly attended by mothers during school time, some of whom found that when all their children had gone to school they had time for themselves – the yoga proved to be an enjoyable salubrious activity. Evening classes were attended by persons from all walks of life including the Coordinator of Covent Garden Opera House, a Homeopath, Nurses, Primary School Teachers, College Lecturers, an Aromatherapist, Waitresses, Builders, Plumbers, an Accountant and last but not least a 79 year old gentleman – veteran and natural comic who frequently had us in stitches.

Each ROUCF yoga session was organised so that the Trainer's classes would steadily progress at the same pace. Each session would include Salutation, Breathing, warming-up-movements, Yoga Postures (Asanas), Mindfulness, Sense Withdrawal, Visualization, Yoga Theory and Relaxation. In addition, Sri Paul included in ROUCF 10 preparations to deepen concentration, attention and awareness during the practice of Asanas. These were:

1. RELAX THE BODY before, during and especially after exercise.

2. VISUALIZE THE ASANA in full like a television picture.

3. TALK TO THE MUSCLES which will be used in the Asana.

4. BREATH AND MOVEMENT COORDINATION to cultivate a working harmony within the body.

5. BRAIN AND BODY COORDINATION – Having awareness of the first thoughts followed by the action is good for discipline. Observation of this thought-action process helps develop concentration.

6. PHYSICAL OBSERVATION – Observing the physical state is a 'feeling' visualisation that should be done before, during and after practice of Asana.

7. OBSERVE YOURSELF PSYCHOLOGICALLY – Turning within to develop an awareness of the psychological state and by observing the same one can learn how to control it.

8. CHECK YOUR MOOD BEFORE STARTING ASANA – If your mood is good your body will respond in a similar fashion. Change your mood for the better by the process of thinking and acting. Tell yourself to feel love and compassion and be grateful for love.

9. DEDICATE YOUR ASANA TO THE COSMIC UNIVERSE in a spirit of thankfulness.

10. IDENTIFICATION – I am the Cosmic Universe in miniature and I recognise my unlimited abilities and desires only to complete my mission successfully on this earth and then return to my place of origin – the Cosmic Universe. A really delightful system of yoga!

Gypsy Caravan

A friend of mine, Ernest, introduced me to country life. Until then I had spent most of my time in London and was now about to experience the beginning of another new phase in my life. I found that the colour green is very good for the eyes – it helps to relax, soothe and refresh them. I found myself looking for the first time at the green countryside all around me and, among other things, saw the intricacy of perfection in form. I stayed in my friend's Bow-Top gypsy caravan, on a plot of land owned by some of his friends.

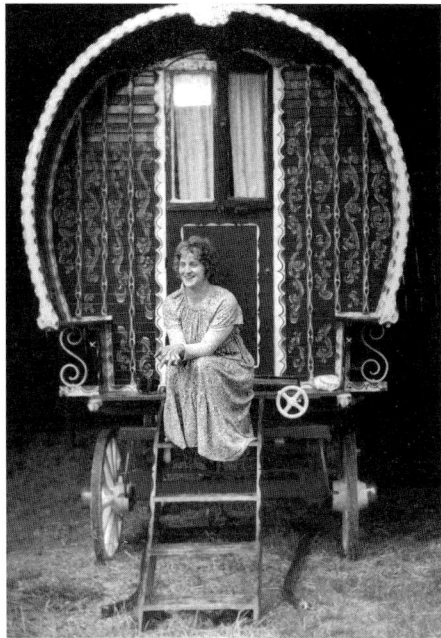

The owners of the plot of land where the caravan was sited became very good friends and when Ernest wanted to sell his gypsy caravan I decided to buy it. The owners of the land, Valerie and David Tarbuck, agreed that I could keep it parked on their land, and stay any time I wished. For my part, I agreed that they could use the caravan to put up friends whenever I was not there. Almost every other weekend I travelled from the concrete jungle, London, to the Kent countryside and stayed in my gypsy caravan. The most remarkable thing about the caravan was that there was enough floor space inside to do my yoga practice, even though most of the postures involved standing, sitting and lying on the floor. I would sit usually cross-legged in front of the door entrance, and meditate on the greenness of the surrounding countryside. This to me was like a foretaste of heaven!

Valerie and David had a very wide circle of friends. They too had once lived in London and entertained many visitors throughout the summer, so I was able to socialise, if I pleased, in their 'open house'. This time of my life was most liberating. In fact both Valerie and David virtually adopted me and really helped me through the last stages of my recuperation period from the car accident. I learnt from them that LOVE always wins and that we can love ourselves and alter our lives to be more harmonious and joyful! This is our true and natural entitlement in life if we so choose it to be!

After Grove Park Yoga Centre

As my father's business expanded, my use of his hayloft had to cease, so I moved to a hired room above a travel agent. Unfortunately it was a small stuffy room and very hot in the summer. Soon after this the numbers in the classes diminished along with my interest. I was being drawn back to the country where there was plenty of space and fresh air.

I had the opportunity to move into the depths of the country and took my Bow-Top caravan to Carmarthenshire, to a piece of land adjacent to a cottage which I could use for domestic purposes during the cold weather. I also had the opportunity to hold a small yoga group in Martin and Kathy Holyoak's farmhouse in a small hamlet named Maesllyn. In response to a notice placed on the local newsagent's noticeboard, six people joined me to form a group which met one evening a week for eighteen months. This proved to be a rich experience for us all. We shared our experiences, philosophies and beliefs, had lots of fun during our yoga sessions and the group became dynamic. We gained much from each other's interests and experiences – beyond yoga practice – and I found I gained a greater understanding of humankind, as did, I'm sure, the other members of the group.

The beginning of my Yoga work in Special Needs

Financial considerations took me to London again, where I was fortunate to literally walk into a newly created job teaching yoga at the SELTEC College for Adults, in Lewisham (academic year 1978–79). Initially, this involved a lunchtime yoga session for students and staff which was tremendously popular – within three weeks fifty people had enrolled for the class. At the end of the third session a Special Needs tutor, Leslie Seal, came up and asked me if I had ever worked with people with learning difficulties (labelled educationally sub normal (ESN) in those days). I said that I hadn't. She asked if I would like to visit her group in the Special Needs department of the college, to see if I thought her students could follow the yoga practices.

I welcomed the idea. Having a special needs background myself, I had discovered from the numerous yoga techniques I had practised, that regular practice undoubtedly uplifts and enlivens anyone who participates, let alone a disabled person, provided that the techniques are suitable and within their competence. So the next day I visited Leslie's class to meet the group of six teenagers. I liked the friendly way the group was working together to cover basic life skills and I agreed to do a trial period, with a college contract, to see if yoga would be suitable for these students.

During the first six weeks I thought we were going nowhere as there seemed to be little evidence that the students were learning anything. Then, at the beginning of the session just after half-term, one of the students said, 'Look at me' as she was doing the 'Full Butterfly' technique that we had previously practised together. Later on another student who only had two fingers on each hand, showed me how she could do the alternate nostril breathing using one finger of each hand alternately. At last I was getting an active response.

I learned from this group that such persons have a head start with what is needed to accept yoga, simply because ideally we have to learn to love, to trust, and to have faith in ourselves, and these marvellous people have such a hunger for loving attention.

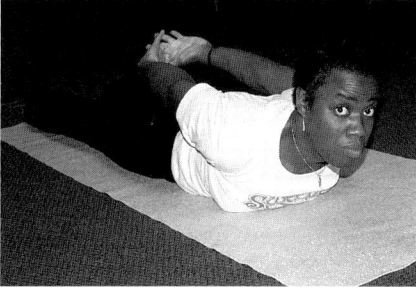

The student from this group whose face was used for the YOU & ME logo.

And I found that this need can be guided into helping each one realise their potential, with the added quality of giving and receiving affection, by encouraging them to love themselves in their mind and body. It is by loving oneself – no matter who or what type of person one may be – that we can conquer fear, and demonstrate our human right to be alive and happy. It is noteworthy that the physical and mindful yoga techniques utilise the non-intellectual aspects of our psyche and develop new areas of consciousness.

On the strength of the sessions at SELTEC College going so well, we were visited by the Head of Special Needs of Southwark Adult Institute, Chris Lloyd, who after watching a session, told me he was very impressed by the students response to the yoga and invited me to work on his Special Needs project at Southwark Institute. This of course, I was eager to do.

The core group

I was pleased I had taken the inspirational advice of a yoga teacher, Robert Hughes, from Hartfield House, Streatham Hill, who had several years experience working with psychiatric patients at Tooting Bec hospital. He told me that it is vital to have an assistant or someone who is well-known to group members so that the early stages of practice for each one are not handicapped by fear. He also recommended the benefit of two 2-hour weekly sessions in a well ventilated spacious room.

To my delight all these requirements were met and the sessions began. This first group at the Institute continued for six years and can be thought of as my 'core' group. I knew there were a lot of yoga practices we could do together, to test their suitability. I kept a record on video of most of these techniques, and in 1983 produced a video of my core group called 'Yoga for Mentally Handicapped Marvellous Human Beings', which I showed in the United Kingdom, India (1984–85), and France (1986), to give inspiration to others.

I found that it was best to keep yoga instructions simple, and to use straightforward language appropriate to the individual's level of understanding. From the yoga exercises, students gained noticeable strength and stamina with improved dexterity and coordination. They were interested in learning about their basic anatomy and physiological functions, and about breathing in and breathing out through either the nose or the mouth – the latter being necessary in the case of some people who physically cannot breathe through their nose. The students were also interested to learn about the connection of the diaphragm with the breath and through their breathing practice they gained an awareness of the wonderful energy and life-force within the body. This work became very interesting and worthwhile for me.

In the early stages, I worked with the core group, holding two classes a week for two hours. We had good conditions for our practice – a well-ventilated, spacious room with a non-slip yoga mat for each of us. I also had the assistance of one member of staff to help me with the students' practice and any problems that might occur during the session. Taking into account that most people with learning difficulties do not take readily to change, you can imagine the challenge we had with this core group who were all in their thirties and for the first time in their lives were being asked to activate their atrophied bodies into new bodily positions of yoga. On top of this, I was unfamiliar to them …

It took quite a while for me to win this groups' confidence and persuade them to move their bodies. Fortunately there was no time restriction. The Head of Special Needs was in favour of yoga being an additional interest in the Southwark Institute's Project for disabled people, so I was allowed to pioneer this work on a trial basis for a considerable time. The introduction of yoga techniques involving some easy breathing, relaxation and chanting gradually started to develop the group's interest and allowed them to explore capabilities which had hitherto lain dormant. Over a period of time, the members progressed physically and mentally at their own pace and in their own way. During the six years I spent working with this group, they blossomed beyond expectation. Not only did they develop more control of their bodies, they became more sensory-aware of different parts of the body and also cultivated their imagination and self-image by visualising being well and happy. Some group members proved capable of guiding the rest through a few simple warming-up movements, yoga postures and breathing, and gave competent instructions for relaxation. Each session finished with everyone chanting, 'One we are one, one we are one, one we are one, all together we are all one'.

By 1983 the students had developed the self-discipline and self-confidence to follow a recording I had made of the yoga instructions, with melodic music playing in the background. Thus while I was on my summer holiday, they were able to continue with this practice in their Daycentre, often with an audience of visitors attending the same centre. The students demonstrated their skills to very good effect and showed great satisfaction in the extent to which they could control their actions through the yoga techniques they had learned. Our practice of mindful techniques helped to awaken their dormant brain potential and from conscious relaxation these students learned how to let go of tensions and hang-ups from disabling past experiences. From this they were able to welcome happiness into their lives, and to look forward to enjoying their burgeoning relationships with their family and friends.

The following is a report on the individuals in this core group and steady progress made through the regular yoga sessions. It was published in the *YOGA for Health* Journal, September/October 1983.

PETER was very competent and devoted to his yoga practice. He disciplines himself to practise every day for up to 4 hours. He has moderate learning difficulties, yet has an incredible memory for famous people, such as film stars, pop stars and their music. Every Tuesday, in preparation for our yoga session, he used to get up at 4.40 a.m. to fit in his yoga practice, before leaving home to make his 5-mile journey on foot to join us at the Daycentre and assist with the yoga session, which he did regularly for the last three years.

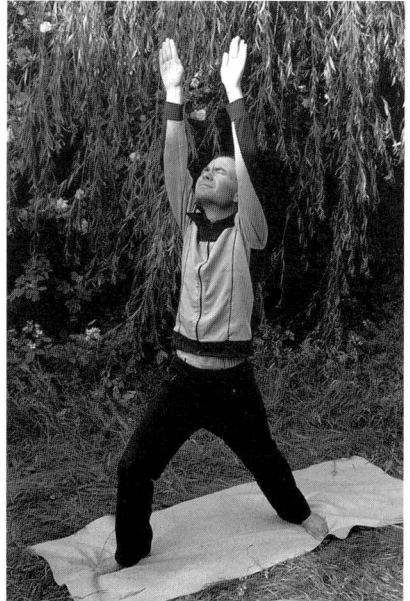

Peter Rands, my assistant.

TINA joined this class in its third year, and proved to be extremely capable in performing postures soon after she joined.

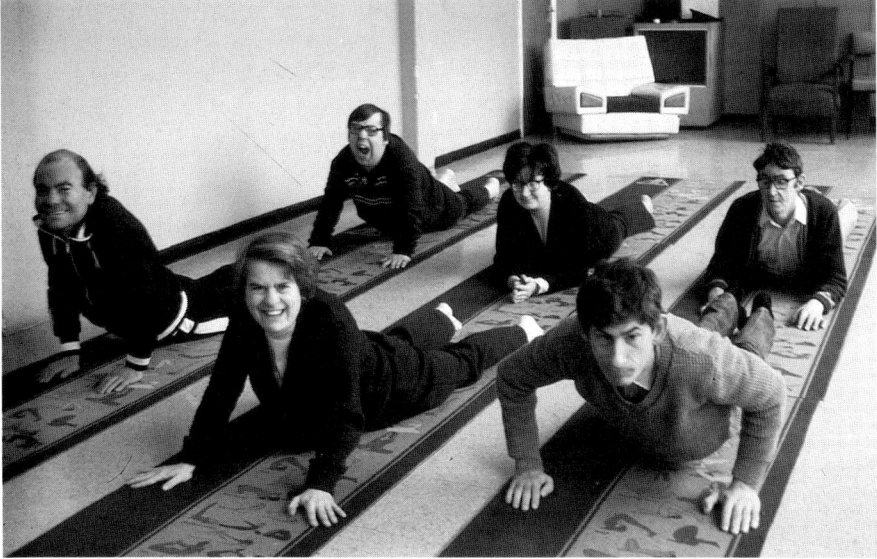

The core group (minus Jean).

JOHN had learning difficulties and defective vision. Sometimes his mind wandered, yet he had learned to follow the yoga instructions and perform the postures well with his agile body. Unfortunately he was a heavy smoker and could not breathe easily through his nose. He had an echolalic speech defect, and after relaxation sessions he would speak about the wonders of nature and repeatedly ask what caused the dew on the grass early in the mornings, what a rainbow was and why did all those colours appear and then disappear again.

JANET had feet which suggested Turner's Syndrome and was very overweight. She was visually impaired, although she did have partial sight, plus she had a moderate degree of deafness. Sometimes she failed to follow instructions. She lacked coordination of movement when she got left behind the others – then she would panic and become all fingers and thumbs. At other times she would manage to keep up with the movement coordinated with the rhythm of the breath. In time Janet learned by heart to instruct the rest of the group in our modified alternate nostril breathing (Sukh Pavak). In fact she had been taught this technique for her own use, so as to balance the right and left sides of her body in correlation to her brain and body coordination.

Janet had slight difficulty in holding up her arms, but over the six years, she had definitely gained the ability to perform the yoga movements, for she was able to raise her arms up high to do the 'Salute to the Sun'. Janet had slowly but surely learned a great deal from the yoga sessions!

DENNIS had cerebral palsy and left hemiplegia. Over the six-year period he progressed by consciously stretching and aligning his mind and body. During the first year of his yoga practice he had not been able to raise his right arm above his shoulders, but he later showed us how he could raise both arms almost straight above his head. Dennis's attributes of endeavour and endurance enabled him to acquire skill and more flexibility in practising his yoga.

JEAN was the one who always liked to be busy. She would help John arrange our yoga mats, and carry them away to be neatly piled after class. She had an over-active solar plexus, and I am sure her practice of diaphragmatic breathing gave her better control of her nervous energy. For fourteen years she suffered with headaches and vomiting, which was diagnosed as 'abdominal migraine', but soon after starting yoga she was free from such attacks apart from occasional slight discomfort. Relaxation sessions especially helped to calm and soothe her mentality; she had poor concentration in class and found relaxation difficult. After all the yoga time spent together Jean would, more often than not, close her eyes, whereas in the early days they would be darting all over the place! Over the six years she began to reach a fine state of relaxation and became more at peace with herself.

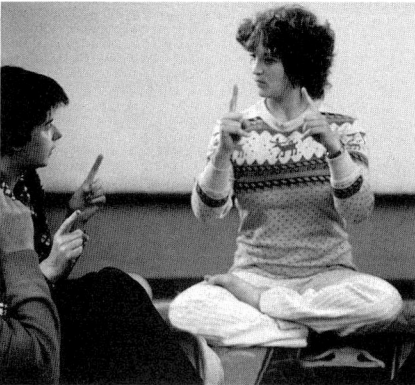

Jean (left), the remaining member of the core group, with myself.

ALAN was registered blind and although he could see a little close-to, he saw double and one of his eyes had rotary movement. He had many operations for cataracts. Alan had swollen feet and became wobbly if he took one foot off the floor. After a couple of years, with his enthusiasm to get to the hall, he would run in front of the rest of us to get there first! He became more active and sprightly from his regular yoga practice. Although his sternum was depressed, he had developed control over his breath, through keeping in time with the instructions. On occasions Alan took the yoga class, and coherently spoke the exact words he had learned to instruct the group in some warming-up movements which other members enjoyed following!

During my second year working with this group, I was informed that my qualification from ROUCF was not recognised by the Inner London Education Authority (I.L.E.A.), so I did a further 2-years training for the British Wheel of Yoga Diploma. As part of this 2-year diploma, I attended many practical and theoretical seminars in addition to my weekly yoga classes. I found there were many other yoga schools such as Satyananda, Vivekananda, Sivananda, F.R.Y.O.G. Yoga, Albion Yoga Movement and the Yoga for Health Foundation. All the classes I attended were different from each other. Naturally, I preferred those teachers whose approach and personality was not abrupt and too vigorous, especially since I had to be careful with my neck.

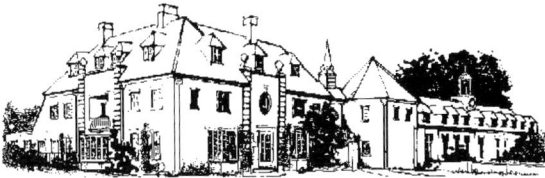

Ickwell Bury, the Yoga for Health Foundation's residential centre.

I regularly visited the Yoga for Health Foundation at their magnificent residential centre at Ickwell Bury, Bedfordshire to attend various seminars with Howard Kent and other eminent visiting yoga teachers. A particularly outstanding teacher was Malcolm Strutt, who covered the psychological aspects of yoga. This practical weekend seminar added a new aspect to my yoga education and several years later this led to the conclusion of the colour-coding in the YOU & ME system. During his seminar, Malcolm introduced me to the seven levels of consciousness and the significance of the spectrum colours in relation to the different colour vibrations of the seven chakra – vortices of energy – centres in the body.

At this time, I made friends with an Italian lady called Lucy and we decided that we wanted to learn more from Malcolm. We arranged to attend his Centre for Conscious Living, in Chippenham, for an intensive 2½-day course covering the more theoretical aspects of the seven coloured levels of consciousness and yoga. This study with Malcolm reinforced what we had learnt from him at Ickwell Bury, and he also introduced us to 'Mantra Yoga' – the science of sound and vibration. We chanted several sounds – mainly the sounds 'A', 'U', 'M' – with awareness of the sound vibrations affecting different areas of the body. When these three sounds are joined together they become 'OM' – a well-known ancient Sanskrit sound that can create calmness of mind, steadiness of thought and preparation for meditation. This in turn benefits the mind, emotions and health.

Later that night, upstairs in the loft where Lucy and I were staying, we did a little meditation sitting on the floor between our two beds before we said good night and went to bed. Almost immediately we both heard in the distance the 'OM' sound being chanted. At first we thought that it must be Malcolm, but it was rather late, and there was more than one chant at a time, so we weren't sure. In fact, there were several chanting sounds which seemed interminable, with each one starting after another. Bewildered, Lucy and I thought it might have been a cassette playing. But the strange thing was, the sounds were coming from different directions – up through the floor, through the walls, down through the ceiling. The tone of the OM sounds changed from low pitched monk-like sounds to high pitched beautiful angelic sounds. We were aware of the on-going chanting pleasant sound in the background which was calming enough to eventually make us drop-off to sleep at around 2 a.m. Next morning at breakfast, we asked Malcolm about this and he laughed and said he was tucked up in bed asleep by 11.30 p.m.

So far the only explanation for this occurence that I have managed to come up with is that we heard the all pervading OM sound that is said to have been around for centuries. In the words from the bible: 'In the beginning was the Word and the Word was God.' In the same light, the Sanskrit OM sound means to be one with God. We both felt very privileged to have had this unique experience together, otherwise neither of us would have really believed it to have been any more than a dream!

These profound experiences were my initial introduction to the vibration of colour and sound, which resulted, about fourteen years later, in the YOU & ME sound, colour and Whole-Body-Movement system.

After attaining my British Wheel of Yoga Diploma, I decided to further my teaching qualifications with a City and Guilds Teaching Certificate with a core-subject in Special Needs. By its nature Yoga is an area with which you become subjectively involved. Indeed, it can be a challenge to view it objectively. To complete my certificate, I had to try and view the learning process objectively and identify end goal outcomes. This was the start of my coupling the eastern introspective, tangible teachings into a western accountable format. This combination evolved into a western accountable behavioural modification format that resulted, several years later, into the competence-based format YOU & ME training programmes.

Following the car accident, I also became interested in 'Science of Mind' philosophy which is basically the creative power of the mind through positive thinking. This is a practical approach for applying conscious positive thought to everyday experiences. This philosophy teaches that we can choose and determine our own destiny, analogous to the idea of 'the loom weaving different colours and patterns according to thought of the weaver'. The universal spiritual law 'As ye sow, so shall ye reap' applies to both our own experiences and to responses we get from others, and is expressed in a more modern saying 'All the flowers of all our tomorrows lie in the seeds of today.' This is the basis of Karma yoga – the yoga of actively doing good.

In 1982 I joined a metaphysical group in London that was led by a very special lady, Mrs Vereker. She had taken the Science of Mind teaching course under Dr Frederick Bailes, author of 'Your Mind Can Heal You' (1941, reprinted due to popular demand in 1971 and again 1985) and in her retirement devoted most of her time to teaching this universal truth to individuals who came to her seeking help. On Monday evenings her home was open to a group of us who saw some miracles happen as a result of following her teachings. The people attending were surprisingly varied and included a barrister, a doctor, a school principal, a fashion designer, a musician, artists, teachers and business people. My involvement with this group helped me understand the meaning of positivity and goodness. The following is an example of this understanding applied in a real life situation.

Chris Gunstone (folk musician and dance teacher) and I made a professional studio recording entitled 'Yoga for All'. On the tape,

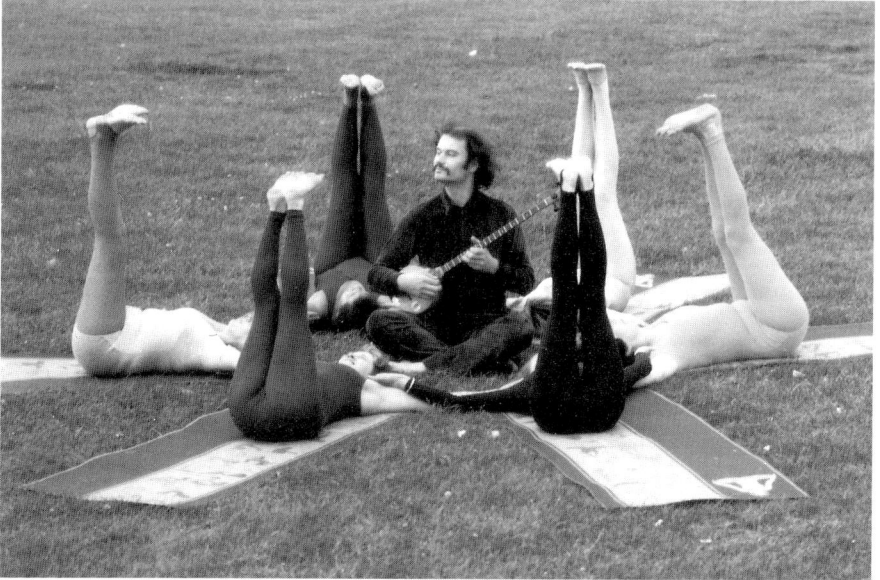

The front cover photograph of the 'Yoga for All' casette.

Chris played his own compositions in time with the breathing rate to my instructions for performing yoga postures. The front cover, sponsored by 'Carita House, Leisure Wear', depicted leotards and track-suit in each of the spectrum colours. Six of us wore them while demonstrating a posture in a circle; Chris wore a violet coloured track-suit and sat in the middle playing a tambura.

Around this time, I had directed a video production at the college television department, showing the seven of us demonstrating the different coloured yoga postures while following the instructions given on the 'Yoga for All' cassette. I planned to use this video at the Olympia exhibition of Mind, Body and Spirit in a couple of weeks' time. It was then that I received a letter from the Vice-Principal asking to see me in his office two days later. Apparently someone had reported to him that I was going to use this video, made with the college's resources, for my own commercial purpose.

At first I was devastated that after several months of preparation and successful filming, the video had been withdrawn by the college until further notice. I consulted Mrs Vereker the day before my meeting with the Vice-Principal. She listened attentively to my story. She was a very clear-thinking, direct and practical lady. I told her that, even though the video had been confiscated, I was hoping to be able to show it on my stall at the Olympia exhibition.

Then, as she started telling me to relate to the Vice-Principal's higher level of understanding, I felt a tremendous surge of energy sweeping across the room and engulfing me. I asked if she could explain it and she smiled and said that every morning when she gets up she goes to her window and opens the curtains and mentally says 'Universe, allow the life force to flow through me so that I can do good work and benefit others.' I realised that I had experienced this source of 'universal energy' which is all around us and which can be tapped into if we but claim it. Well, as expected, the Vice-Principal allowed me to have the video recording with permission to show it at the Olympia exhibition hall, on condition that I did not sell copies of the video – which I had not intended to do anyway. I was allowed to sell the 'Yoga for All' cassette which I had produced in a commercial recording studio and not with college resources. This video was enjoyed by many hundreds of visitors at the exhibition, some of whom saw Hatha yoga being performed for the first time.

Another lesson I learnt from Mrs Vereker was to see all my students as perfect human beings and not to accept anything less. I have carried this lesson with me throughout my work. Of course there have been ups and downs, but I always aim to think positively and consciously and ignore any negativity. This attitude has helped me greatly in my work in special needs where there can be a lot of sadness and frustration if we allow it to affect our consciousness in that way.

Mrs Vereker taught me to know that 'perserverance always gets you there in the end'. Over the past twenty years I have continued to develop the YOU & ME system for people with learning difficulties who generally cannot easily join a mainstream yoga class. I believe I have been granted a second chance – by surviving a serious car accident and overcoming the succeeding traumas through the practice of yoga – and I have found a way that is appropriate and safe to help other disabled peoples' emotional, mental and physical needs, and their personal development. I also believe I have an affinity with these people because of my previous experience of loss of memory and feeling as if I was trapped in my body, unable to easily express myself. This feeling lasted nearly two years and was the most frightening and lonely time imaginable. Now that I have regained my memory, communication, mobility and social skills, I feel able to speak and act on behalf of disabled people who are in a similar position concerning getting around, communicating, expressing and relating with others in their environment.

When Mrs Vereker died the group lost its mainstay, but happily we have kept in touch and occasionally meet up and renew the bond between us. Relationships are all-important in our personal development and human understanding. When we befriend persons with learning difficulties a relationship develops by accepting each other's differences, having a greater understanding of our human nature, and embracing the higher qualities of life, often overlooked, such as appreciation, patience, courage, generosity, modesty and compassion.

Broadening and consolidating my work

I contacted the local Grove Park Hospital for people with learning disabilities, which led to my training three RNMH nurses and five recreational staff, along with eight patients. I was also asked to train members of staff in the Occupational Therapy (OT) department, involving OTs and OT Aides and gave some integrated 'hands on' sessions with various patients. These sessions were appreciated by all. Later, in 1985, the interest this yoga training created led to the video production of 'A Sporting Chance', produced by the British Sports Association, with commentary from pop star Ian Dury. I also trained staff at the Hollies Home in Eltham and gained further employment from Greenwich County Council – Sherard Road Daycentre.

Having personally experienced benefits from the regular practice of yoga, I developed a fervent desire to learn more about it, and to visit India to attend the yoga ashrams and meet the masters about whom I had heard so much. Eventually my wish was fulfilled through winning an award from the Winston Churchill Memorial Trust to go to India to study the therapeutic value of yoga for disabled people. The criteria of the Trust is for its fellows to go abroad to gain knowledge and skills to benefit people in Britain. Due to family circumstances, and my wanting to visit India in the late autumn (after the monsoon), I did not take up my fellowship until almost a year later. Meanwhile, I used the time to prepare for my trip by writing to many organisations and people in the UK and India to ask for help with suitable contacts to enable me to make the most of my visit.

In March 1984, I was able to arrange a meeting with Mr John Hart, Inspector for Special Needs for the Inner London Education Authority, at County Hall. He listened to my story about the core yoga group at Southwark. He agreed that yoga should be made more available in the sphere of education for people with learning difficulties. This meeting actually paved the way for yoga to be accepted as a recognised subject for such people and it also resulted in the in-service training course for yoga teachers in London.

On the strength of my meeting with Mr Hart, Chris Lloyd – the Head of Special Needs for Southwark – agreed to fund my training other yoga teachers to teach yoga to people with learning difficulties in an integrated group, with the core group of six students, at the Southwark Institute. This in-service training started in September 1984 on one full day a week for ten weeks with twelve yoga diploma/student teachers. This training was completed the day before I flew to India in mid-December.

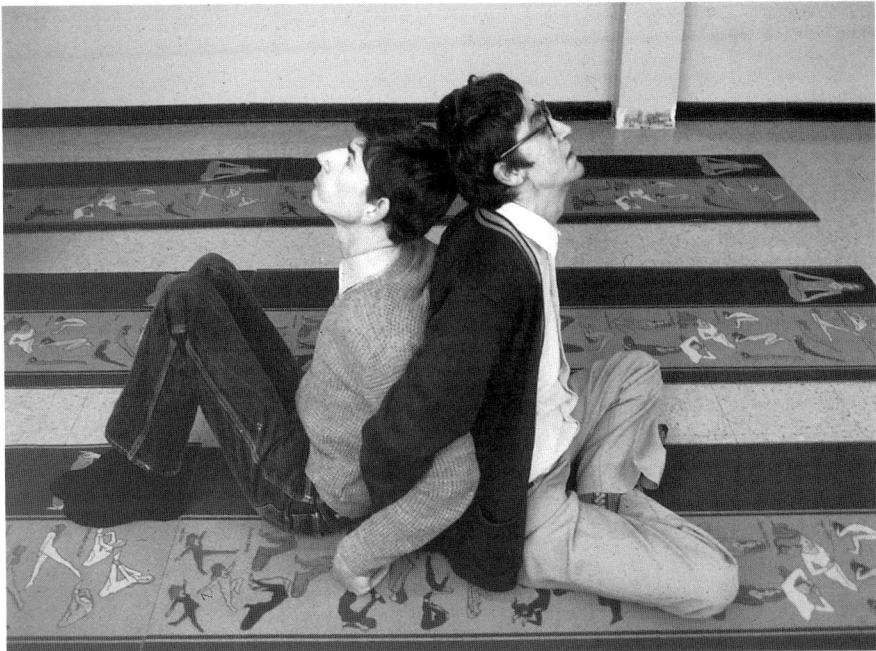

Dennis and John, members of the Core Group, practising their yoga.

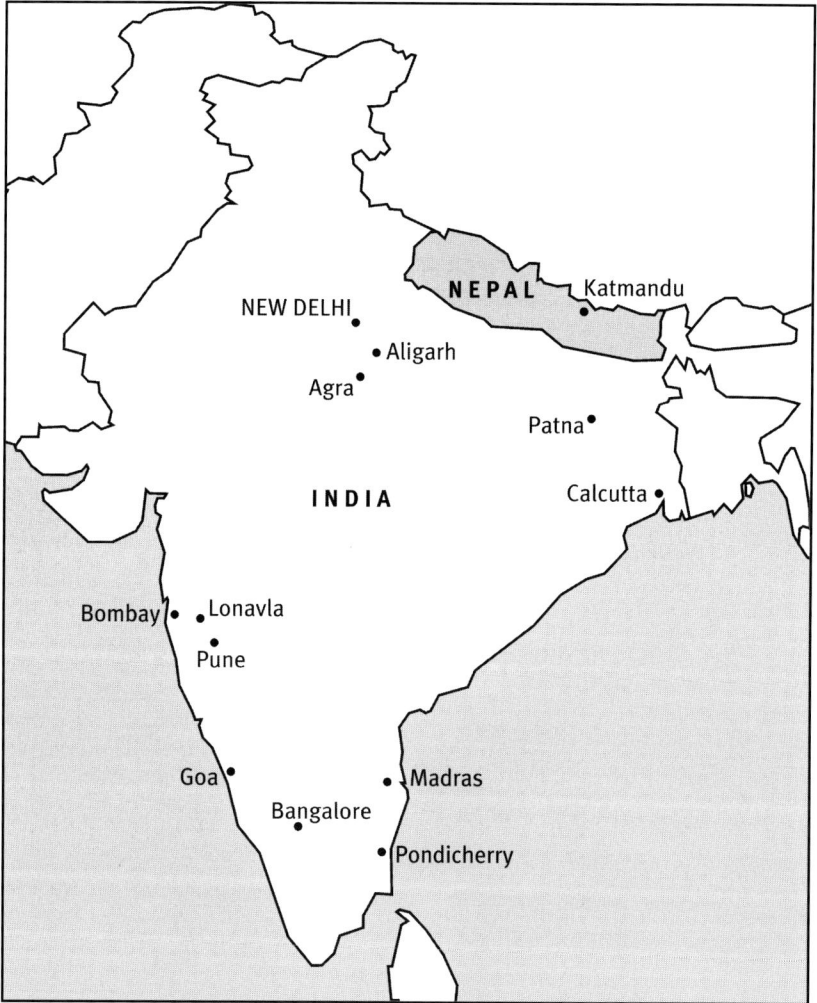

Map to indicate places visited during my Winston Churchill Fellowship.

Part Two

India

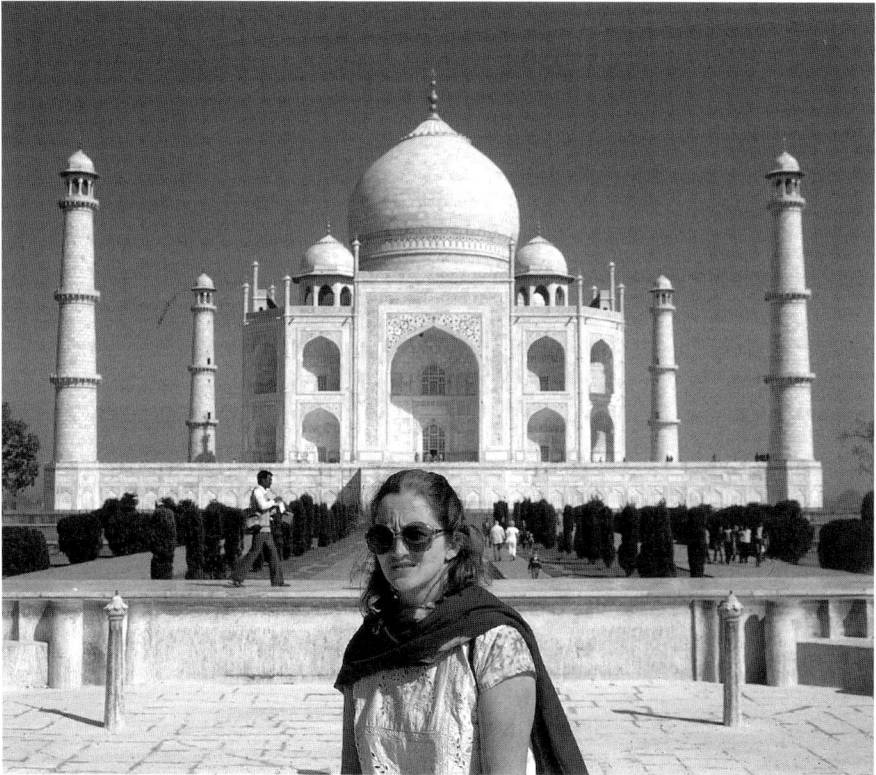

CHAPTER TWO

Investigating the therapeutic value of yoga for disabled people in India

In preparation for my Churchill Fellowship I actually spent eleven months planning and making the necessary arrangements for what was an Indian adventure – studying yoga for disabled people in seven states of India – Haryaha, Maharashtra, Goa, Karnataka, Tamil Nadu, Bihar, and Uttar Pradesh. In December 1984, I left London for Delhi accompanied by Chris Gunstone (by then my fiancee) who supported me throughout my mission. I was able to cope with the tremendous amount of travelling involved by his tireless efforts in doing all the necessary haggling with taxi-drivers, rickshaw-drivers, horse-and-carriage drivers, and even rail and air ticket clerks. Chris carried most of our heavy baggage, including the video and equipment, which I would never have managed on my own.

I arranged to go to the established yoga educational and health research institutions that dealt with the variety of problems experienced by the disabled. I also visited various special education institutes for disabled children and adults. I was privileged to meet some of the greatest yoga masters and teachers as well as special educationalists, medical professionals, and some remarkable disabled people in ashrams, special schools, yoga research institutions, and hospitals. During these meetings Chris diligently filmed the proceedings. All this visual and audio material, depicting the splendid work done for the disabled in India, added greatly to the value of the material I collected and noted down for my report to the Churchill Trust.

In every city we visited we had to get used to the serious air pollution caused by exhaust fumes and from the charcoal-burning stoves which were the chief means of heating. There was constant noise and bustle among the colourfully dressed populace, most of whom were the so-called 'Untouchables'. Many of them lived in squalor, in broken-down shacks with canvas roofing, though a few were slightly better housed. Various languages were spoken in the different states, but luckily those who had received schooling had been taught English, so we were able to communicate very well. Sanskrit words may be spelt differently in the different states so there was variation in the spelling of the Sanskrit names of some of the postures (asanas). Fortunately this difference in spelling does not alter the meaning of the names. During our visit we travelled approximately 6,000 miles, staying mostly at good hotels, ashrams and private homes in which we received wonderful hospitality.

My belief that yoga could be taught by Special Needs staff in schools, colleges, training centres and hospitals, and by carers and parents at home, was confirmed by my research. During my tour I witnessed valuable interdisciplinary teamwork producing individual yoga programmes for children and adults with learning difficulties, for the elderly, and for people who were physically disabled, blind, and/or aurally impaired.

The Churchill Trust requires its Fellows to write a full report at the end of their Fellowship. I put pen to paper and recorded my rich and varied experiences in a 50,000-word report, together with 12 hours of edited video material. I described my experiences at two international yoga conferences (where I was a guest speaker) at Kaivalyadhama, Lonavla and YOCOCEN, Delhi; and at visits to nineteen different centres, hospitals and ashrams in seven Indian states. This report was compiled from the copious notes I took on my travels plus the audio and video recordings. I was grateful for the loan of equipment by Canon UK and British Sports Association for the Disabled.

It was therapeutic for me to recall my Indian adventure – investigating yoga for disabled people. As mentioned, I had suffered loss of memory twelve years before, and for the first time in my life I could call on a wealth of experiences all which were vivid in my memory. These experiences were fascinating to recall and share with others. This opportunity revived my confidence in my memory, particularly as some of my report and video material has since been published.

My Indian Fellowship resulted in many detailed reports and several videos. Some of these reports are included in this book, and others giving in-depth details are available individually. Full details are given at the end of this book.

CHAPTER THREE

Kaivalyadhama –
Yoga Research Institute

An institute for scientific philosophico-literacy research and yoga training. I am most grateful to Howard Kent, Director of Yoga for Health Foundation, Beds., and Dr Robin Monro, Director of Yoga Bio-Medical Trust, London, who both suggested I visit this Institute during my Fellowship.

Swami Kuvalayanada (1883–1966) started the renaissance movement in yoga in 1924, with a vision of integrating yoga into the world of science. He discovered, while performing various yoga practices under the guidance of the Paramhansa Madhavdas of Madras, some very remarkable effects on his body and mind, and he marvelled at the potency of yoga which he was unable to explain in a scientific and rational way. Although spiritually inclined and idealistic, Swami Kuvalayanada was also a strict rationalist. For him, any phenomenon, however miraculous-seeming, had to be capable of explanation on a rational basis. To arrive at such an understanding was a challenge to him, and he began to test India's science of yoga (Bharatiya Yogashastra) through experimental investigation using western modern technology. His research sought to make yoga scientific and to spiritualise science. Today this work is being continued by his followers at Kaivalyadhama.

In December 1984 Swami Digambarji (Director) opened the first International Yoga and Research Conference at Kaivalyadhama with the following words: 'Swami Kuvalayanada's goal was to bring the science of yoga to people in a manner that would benefit humanity. He felt the time had come for science and spirituality to play their role together in stabilising societies. This could only be achieved at a point in time where spirituality from the East and science from the West could be brought together. May the Almighty bless us with the wisdom to understand the path for the future development in the field of yoga, so that the light kindled by Swami Kuvalayanada can be kept burning always for the benefit of humanity.'

The conference was attended by scientists, doctors and yoga practitioners from Australia, Sweden, Spain, Germany, Italy,

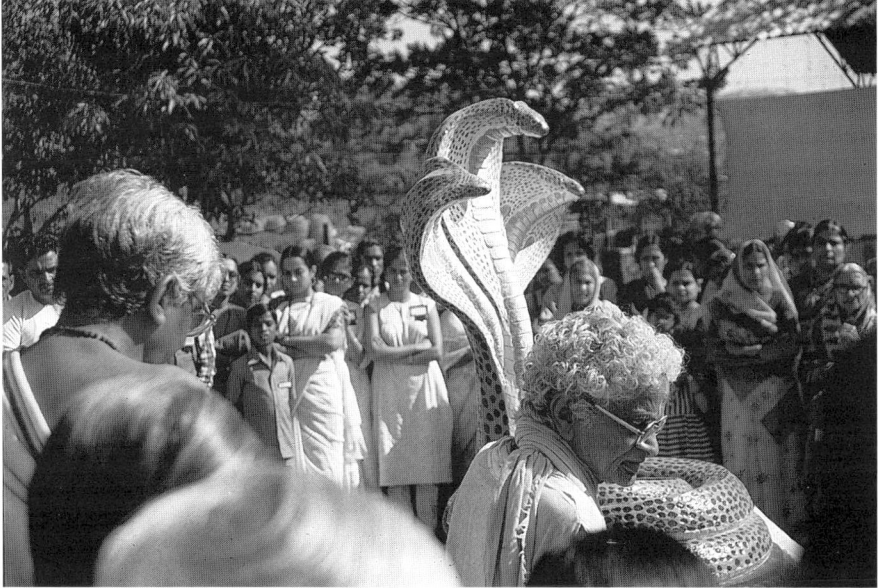
Swami Digambarji conducts the opening ceremony of the conference.

Mexico, Brazil, USA, Britain and India. The delegates and the Kaivalyadhama research team gave inspiring lectures on such subjects as:

- Yoga – a process of education
- The effect of yogic training on some aspects of psychomotor performance
- The effect of yogic training on endurance and flexibility levels
- Shankhaprakshalana (cleansing the body)
- Physiology and yoga
- Integrated approach of yogic therapy for bronchial asthma – a review
- Practical aspect of yoga therapy in cases of bronchial asthma
- Effect of yoga therapy in cases of diabetes and obesity
- Influence of yoga therapy on serum lipase activity in diabetes
- Skin, stress and yoga
- Executives and yoga

- Yoga and Naturopathy
- The rationale of yogic perceptions
- Yoga and correction of criminal behaviour: A pilot study
- Effect of selected yogic practices on blood sugar level of the diabetic patient
- Effect of yoga therapy on obesity and lipid profile
- Possibilities of Jnana yoga therapy for psychosomatic diseases
- Psychotherapy and group yoga
- Use of hierarchy of adopted yoga methods for anxiety in groups of hospitalised patients
- Effect of yogic practices performed in a state of meditation on adolescent anxiety and certain personality variables
- Meditation for better living
- Emotional stability and postures
- Sympathicotonia in diseases and therapy through yoga and related manipulations
- Spinal disorders and yoga therapy
- Neuromotor developmental criteria for item difficulty of yogasanas of spastic disorder
- Preliminary investigations in the use of yoga therapy for ophthalmic disorders
- Utility of yoga for the aged blind – A pilot study.

I was pleased to give a talk on – Yoga for people with learning difficulties, and I showed a video of my core yoga groups' practice.

I was surprised to learn that very few members of my audience had ever considered the suitability of yoga for people with learning difficulties/disabilities. Seeing the skills my core group gained from regular practice convinced them of the appropriateness of yoga for this clientele.

After my talk, Dr Swami Gitananda, Dr Salam, and Mr Vora told me how pleased they were to hear how yoga was benefiting disabled people in the UK. To my delight they each invited me to visit them and observe how they were using yoga as a therapy. I report later on these three worthwhile visits and also on a fascinating meeting I had at the Conference with the elderly Baba Prithwi Singh Azad.

I was very pleased to attend the first International Yoga and Research Conference at Kaivalyadhama. It seems that there is a growing rapprochement between science and yoga which may yet bring to pass what yogis predicted centuries ago – that yoga can redirect the course of both individual and global evolution.

Dr Gharote, Co-Principal of the G.S. College of Yoga and Cultural Synthesis at Kaivalyadhama, said to me, 'Yoga in this day and age needs to be rationally understood to overcome any misconception and mystery behind it'. He wrote in his book 'Guidelines for Yogic Practices' – 'The discipline of yoga passed through several stages, and in course of time different people emerged and a variety of techniques were evolved. Every school of yoga concentrated on specific practices, but the aim remained the same, namely to control the processes of mind. Some of the schools use techniques that deal with the mind directly, and some use indirect means through the body to tackle the mental processes. For the common man the approach to the mind through the body is easier and within his limits; therefore practices which emphasise the use of the body are much favoured.

Practical Hints on the Practice of Yoga

1. All yoga practices should begin with quiet sitting with closed eyes.

2. In the early stages all asana (physical postures) may be performed under the pattern of normal breathing, unless for some reason it is advisable to change this and resort to some special mode of breathing in particular circumstances.

3. It is advantageous to direct the mind to different parts of the body where sensations are felt.

4. Practice of Shavasana (Lying supine relaxing) at intervals during the session of yogic practices is helpful.

5. When practice is performed, the stomach should be empty or only lightly filled.

6. Kriyas (cleansing techniques) and Pranayama (breath control) are better learnt first under proper guidance before being practised on one's own.

7. Regularity in practice is more important than duration.

8. When there is a considerable break in yogic practice it is advisable to start again with a simple exercise.

9. The combination of other exercises with yogic practices can be advantageous, but the two sessions should be kept apart.

10. Moderation is the watchword in yoga, and is applicable to exercise as well as diet.

In my Report I give full explanations of the different types of yoga practices – Asana, Pranayama, Bandhas and Mudras, Kriyas, Meditation and some of the tests carried out in the Research Departments, the Training Dept. and Yogic Hospital. This is accompanied by a 45-minute video 'Scientific Research into Yoga'. From all the yoga masters I was privileged to meet, in nineteen different organisations in India, I learnt that no yoga posture can be regarded beneficial for a particular condition without the toning up of all the bodily systems. Furthermore, I learnt that no particular posture is prescribed for a specific complaint, but that a group of postures should always be used. Thus, the whole person, not just the complaint, is treated. Dr Gharote, Co-Director, of Kaivalyadhama provided me with scientific evidence of this when taking me around the Kaivalyadhama Research Department. This department comprises six sections: Physical Education, Physiological, Electrological, Psychological, Radiological and Biological sections.

The Physical Education section works for health and physical fitness through yoga. Physical fitness factors being researched included: strength, flexibility, stamina, endurance, balance and equilibrium.

The Physiological section studies the effects of yoga on the body. Tests are carried out to observe how the body functions while the student performs a particular exercise.

The Electrophysiological section uses electrographic devices, some of which are among the most advanced technical equipment used in the medical world today, to investigate how the functions of the inner body respond during the practice of yogic techniques. At the time of our visit there was a recently installed sophisticated Polygraph machine which measured the activity of the brain, the heart, the muscles, the respiration, and the temperature. One of these functions was selected and measured by connecting the electrodes of the polygraph to the patient while he performed a particular exercise.

The Psychological section tested many healthy people as well as patients. Investigations were made into the psychological changes, especially concerning emotional stability. Results were very encouraging and showed how psychological attitudes were positively

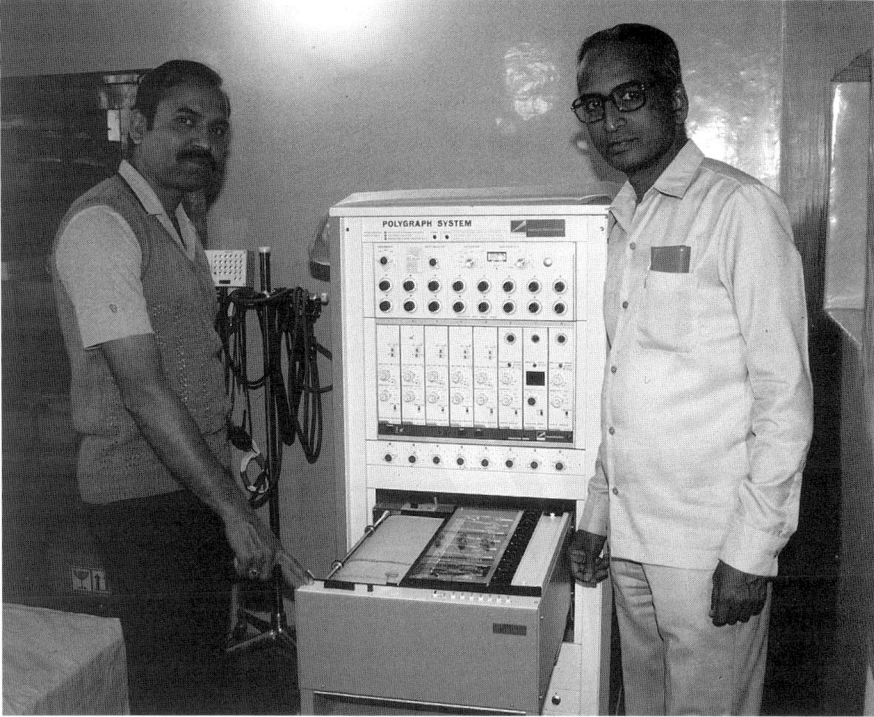

Dr Gharote (right) and colleague standing beside the sophisticated Polygraph machine.

changed through the practice of yoga. The majority of subjects who received yoga treatment eradicated many of their social problems and this brought a new balance and stability to their lives.

The Radiological section uses X-rays to test the effects of various yoga practices, such as the effects of breathing exercises on the respiratory system, and of cleansing techniques to the digestive and eliminatory systems

The Biochemical section uses chemicals to test for biochemical reactions. For example, a seven-week course of yogic treatments was given to diabetic people to test the influence of yoga practice (involving postures, breath control and cleansing techniques) on serum lipase activity. Tests showed a significant reduction in serum lipase activity. This reduction could help to maintain a proper concentration of circulating free fatty acids and could further regulate the insulin level. Quite fascinating!

Address:

Kaivalyadhama Yoga Research Institute, Prabhat Colony, LONAVLA, Bombay – 410 403

CHAPTER FOUR

Encounter with Baba Prithwi Singh Azad – veteran revolutionary

After an intensive day of lectures, Chris and I queued, along with several hundred scientists and yoga enthusiasts, for our evening meal of curry. We shared a table with an elderly gentleman of vigorous appearance, and started chatting to him. We both immediately felt the warmth of his personality and the atmosphere of dynamic goodwill that he generated. He told us that he did not usually eat such highly spiced food – 'rajasic food' as he called it – but followed a careful wholesome and natural diet of 'sattvic foods' which were of much greater benefit to the body. Because of this, and his yoga disciplines, he had succeeded the previous year (1983) in winning the World Veteran Sports Championships at St Johns and gaining four gold medals 'for the honour of my country' at the age of 93! He went on to tell us a fascinating story which, with his permission, we recorded. It was backed up by a long article about him in a communist journal of 1938, a copy of which he showed, and later gave to us. It appeared that he had been a leading revolutionary during the British Raj. He had been greatly respected by Gandhi, who, while disapproving of his methods, nevertheless said of him, 'I would love to have men like this as fellow-pilgrims in the pilgrimage to the temple of freedom'.

Prithwi Singh (as he was then known) was imprisoned, put in chains, and kept in solitary confinement in a small cell. He realised that it was up to him to maintain his health, strength and mental aptitudes, and he recalled the yoga teaching he had received from Swami Vive-

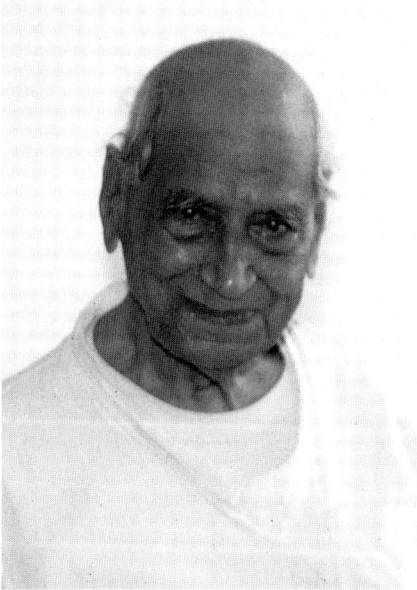

Baba Prithwi Singh Azad.

kananda in the Punjab some years earlier. He did the physical exercises necessary to keep his body strong and supple along with yoga breathing exercises which he found enabled him to assimilate the abominable food served to the prisoners. Food that had a detrimental effect on the health of most of the inmates.

In protest against the brutality with which the prisoners were treated, Prithwi Singh went on a 5-month hunger strike and his weight dropped from 160 to 90 lbs. Force feeding was carried out and severe punishments were inflicted on the rebellious prisoners of whom he was the ringleader.

Later, while being transferred by rail to another jail, he leapt off the moving train, injuring his spine and both knees and breaking his left arm. Despite these injuries, and the chains that still bound him, he managed to walk through the night for several hours before he was recaptured. Later still, he was transferred a second time and again jumped off the train. This time he was uninjured and he made good his escape. He was able to settle down in the Indian countryside and earn his living as a physical culturist, training young men in gymnastics, and instilling into them a spirit of nationalism. No one knew his real identity, and he was loved and admired by those he taught and by the other local inhabitants.

After some years had elapsed, Prithwi Singh decided that he could no longer continue to live in this quiet fashion, completely frustrated and cut off from his main purpose in life of fomenting insurrection against the British. He came out of hiding and gave himself up to the authorities (who had long assumed he must be dead.) He was again put in prison, but eventually, when the situation in India changed, he was released.

Throughout all these times of stress, hardship and suffering, he remained in good health thanks to his regular practice of yoga. Prithwi Singh was unable to do the full yoga postures because of his injuries – in particular his broken left arm had left him with what he described as a 'helping hand' instead of a true hand – but he continued to do his own special system of modified yoga exercises which were within his capabilities, and kept up the yoga breathing.

Prithwi Singh emphasised to us the inestimable benefit to be derived from yoga and the ease with which it can be performed: 'You don't need any apparatus, you don't need much space or time, you don't need any companion. You can perform the exercises on your bed, and 10–20 minutes are all the time that is required. This will keep your limbs agile, improve circulation, and purify the blood. The aim is to breath as deeply as is comfortably possible, but a person who is pursuing spiritual development is in the right state to benefit from yoga breathing even if the air is not pure. The yoga student must understand physiology and the workings of the human body, and must discipline himself to correct eating at the right intervals, and for the right amount of sleep. He must at all times observe himself and be aware of his body and how it is responding. If he ceases at any time to use his body correctly, he should realise this at once and be able to rectify it. The final achievement in yoga is of course the asana Sirshasana – standing on your head – which flushes and recharges the whole system. I cannot practice it myself because my "helping hand" is not strong enough to support me, but the numerous other exercises I perform, together with the breathing and yoga foot massage, have developed me to a pitch where no one in the world can compete with me as Veteran World Athletics Champion!'

We could but marvel and agree! We felt that this splendid old man was an example to us all of what yoga can achieve in overcoming severe obstacles and handicaps.

CHAPTER FIVE

Dr Abdul Salam who instigated a study programme, with Kaivalyadhama and the NAB Lions Home for the Aging Blind

D r Salam told me he was born in 1940 in a remote village in Kanyakumari District, at the southernmost tip of India. At the age of twelve he had to face the onset of retinitis pigmentosa and had to accept this disability in a traditional Indian society. This was in addition to family difficulties arising from his father's death when he was only four, and his mother's deafness caused by breaking her tympanum when banging her head against a wall in an extremity of grief. Dr Salam remained at school until he was seventeen when he had to leave because of increasing blindness and the lack of adequate information about facilities for the education of blind people.

A new life presented itself to Dr Salam when he met Shri E.V. Joseph, another blind man, who inspired him to learn braille. He acquired a tape recorder, type writer and joined college. The struggle for survival afforded him new hope, enabling him to attain an academic record, to acquire a Doctorate in Linguistics, and to obtain gainful employment for a normal productive life. He started work organising self-help programmes for the blind, as well as education and creative opportunities for the weaker sections of society, particularly handicapped people.

In an interview he told me, 'My mother tongue is Tamil, and I speak eight other languages – Malayalam, Kannada, Marsthi, Hindi, English, German, Arabic and Esperanto. I have travelled through different parts of India speaking to handicapped people and preaching the message 'Handicapped people are not only normal human beings, but first-class citizens who should prove their normality by struggle for betterment through self-confidence and self-help.' My work has taken me abroad to Sri Lanka, West Germany, Belgium, the Netherlands, Luxembourg, France, Switzerland, the United Kingdom, Denmark, Sweden, Finland and Norway.

Dr Abdul Salam   35

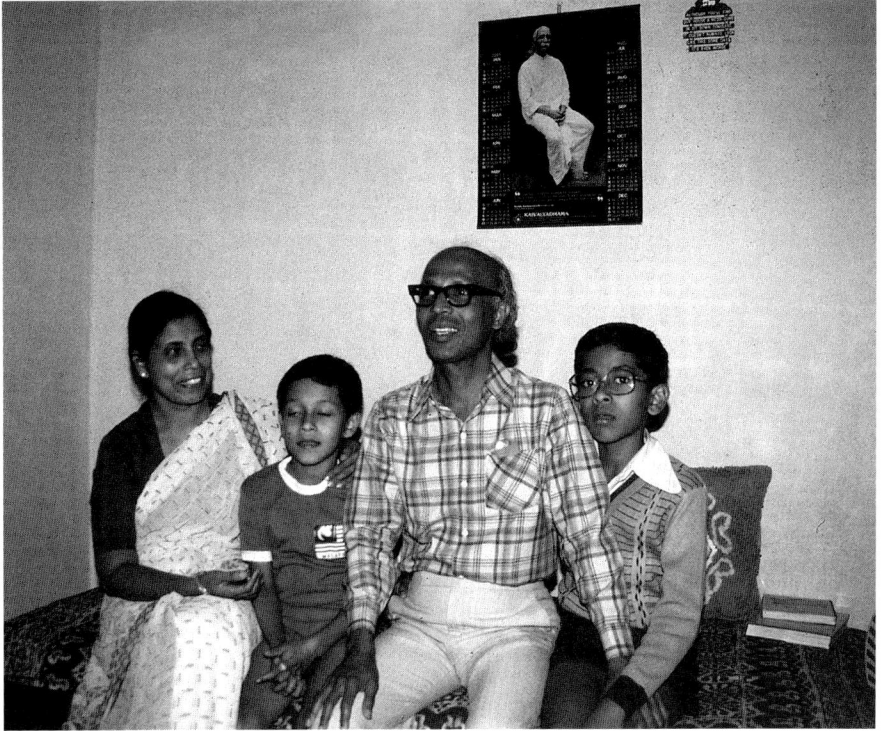

Dr Abdul Salam and his family.

'The use of my white cane makes me mobile. I think a blind person minus mobility is below normal, so I am propagating the use of the white cane everywhere I go. I have chosen to wear glasses, even though I am totally blind, purely for cosmetic reasons, to minimise the disturbance to other people caused by the 'wandering' of my eyes.

'In 1971 I crossed religious and communal boundaries; although my religious background is Muslim, I married Gracy, a teacher who comes from a Catholic family. We have two sons, Mischad who is twelve, and Remi who is seven, and we all lead a very happy and normal family life together. I believe a handicapped person should be free to choose their partner, so that both can pull together for a happy life. I am against the idea that a handicapped person should only marry another handicapped person.

'In my desire to help my handicapped brethren, I endeavoured for a decade and a half to work for their upliftment in a private capacity, but finally accepted employment on behalf of the physically disabled as Officer on Special Duty, Directorate of Social Welfare, Maharashtra State.'

In 1983 the Government of Maharashtra conferred a State Award on Dr Salam as Outstanding Handicapped Employee. In 1984 he explored the idea of a yoga study programme for aging blind men, aimed at finding out how far yoga could help them in their existing living conditions. He said, 'I personally had practised yoga over the past 1½ years, and there is no doubt that my health improved in consequence. I now find that if I don't practise for two consecutive days, I don't feel so healthy or fully active. In fact, before I started yoga I experienced a lot of fatigue and my body felt burdensome, but now I practise for an hour each day and I feel rejuvenated. I was personally taught by Dr Bhole (M.B.B.S., M.D.) from the Kaivalyadhama Yoga and Research Institute, where he has investigated yoga therapy and measured students' progress for several years.

'I asked Dr Bhole if he would accompany me to the NAB Lions Home for the Aging Blind, Khandala, Lonavla, to give an informal introductory talk on yoga so that the inmates could decide for themselves about a yoga programme. He willingly agreed. After his talk, he asked the inmates to experience their breathing. Some of them protested, 'but we don't know we are breathing'. Twenty five inmates decided to take part, and the superintendent, Shri Joshi gave his consent to the programme taking place at the Home. A project proposal entitled 'Yoga for the Handicapped' was then drawn up and sent to the Government, who accepted it and authorised an experimental study for a period of one year, in collaboration with Kaivalyadhama.

'Medical experts from Kaivalyadhama, including Dr Bhole and Clinical Psychologist Mrs Oak, undertook a systematised analysis with scientific assessment of the yogic practices performed by the inmates. The following report on the results was submitted by Dr Bhole to the Maharashtra State Government, India.'

The Problems of Teaching

Generally the most effective method of teaching yoga is to actually demonstrate the technique to the student. Of course, this cannot apply to blind students. Therefore an alternative method of communication had to be worked out quickly.

It was also realised that speech would not be of much use, since some of the participants had become blind in early childhood and therefore had very limited associative memory. Others who had become blind at a later date were comparatively poorly educated and came from the lower strata of society where yoga was hardly ever discussed. Most of the time these people had to struggle for existence, and had no time, place, energy or money to spend on the finer, subtler and higher aspects of human life. In addition, many of the older individuals were partially deaf, so that getting through to them was even more of a challenge.

The various participants were unable to follow any one language like Hindi or Marathi. Because of their background, the usual examples could not be used to communicate with them, as meaning conveyed through words requires previous association – lacking in the case of many of the blind participants.

Developing Teaching Methods for the Physically Handicapped

Individuals that have a physical handicap like blindness or deafness are, of course, perfectly capable of experiencing sensations in the body such as pain, pressure, stretching, compression, getting out of breath, etc. Therefore, this was thought to be the best method of imparting yoga techniques to these students. In the same way, it is usually found that if there is a disability in relation to one of the sense organs like the eye or the ear, the other sense organs acquire extra power in compensation. Blind people have a good sense of touch and hand manipulation. Therefore the following guidelines to educate them were developed in the first week.

Experiencing and Finding Out One's Own Breathing Pattern

This technique was used to experience breathing movements with the help of their own hands on different parts of the body. These movements were compared with the movements of the other inmates and the teacher. Through these experiences they were brought to an appreciation that the nature of breathing movements differed in different individuals, even though the physical structures were similar in them all. Participants were also made to think about the factors responsible for breathing movements and the importance of breathing in comparison with the functions of different organs (which may get disturbed or lost, and thus result in some form of physical disability). Through rational thinking and reasoning, anyone can be convinced of the vital importance of breathing for health and of the ability to manipulate it with a view to enhancing the quality of one's life. The students were asked to consider what should be the correct pattern of breathing in any individual, and why this pattern might become disturbed.

By means of these procedures of experience-cum-thinking-cum-discussion with the participants, the theory of Prana (vital life force), Pranic activity, and its responsibility for breathing and various functions of the body was explained, and the foundation for further instruction in yoga was laid down. This also helped to arouse the interest of the participants and encouraged their voluntary participation in the programme with positive motivation. Even though everybody could appreciate the nature of correct breathing movements, no one was in fact breathing correctly and they were all anxious to have their breathing pattern corrected. As explained earlier, simple asanas were introduced to the class through verbal instruction and the stressing of inner experience. The following examples will throw light on the nature of the instructions given:

Giving Instructions in Asanas (Yoga Postures)

A. Standing on both legs: In this position students were asked to put equal weight on both legs and to be aware of the sensation. They were then asked to distribute their weight equally from the toes to the heels, whilst again experiencing the sensation.

B. Chakrasana (lateral bending). While standing, students were asked to lift the right arm above the head, experiencing the movement of the hand throughout. They were then asked to stretch the hand upwards in such a way that they could experience the whole of the right side of the body from fingertips to toes. While doing this, the left side of the body had to be kept completely relaxed. Maintaining the inner experience, they were told to bend the body to the left in such a way that they would experience stretching on the right side and relaxation on the left. While they did this, the weight on both feet had to remain the same. Finally they were asked to experience the breathing movements – especially on the right and left sides of the chest and of the abdomen – and through this experience they were made to realise the influence of asanas (in this case Chakrasana) on breathing.

After experiencing breathing for a short time – say three to four breaths – they were instructed to straighten the body and bring the right hand down. At the end, any residual tension remaining had to be released by making suitable gross movements or subtle adjustments, as seemed best to the student.

C. Two or three simple asanas were introduced every day, and the students were encouraged to appreciate the effect of each asana on breathing movements. Awareness of the body was experienced in the form of stretching, with bearable discomfort in different areas, according to the constitution and physical condition of the individual. Through this, the asanas helped to release tension and bring about relaxation.

D. Shavasana (corpse posture) was given at the end of the session as follows: Lying prone, become aware of the body without any physical movement. This helped students to recognise areas of tension, which could be released by making gross movements or subtle adjustments so as to get a uniform experience of the whole body. Experiencing the breathing, and extending the sensation all over the body by relaxing various parts. Students were encouraged to differentiate between breathing movements in and out of the body, and the energy responsible for the physical movement of breathing experienced deep within oneself.

Imparting Instructions in Pranayama Breathing

E. The participants were shown how to experience correct breathing with the help of different asanas. Most of them were able to feel the expansion of the body during inhalation, and its shrinking during exhalation.

F. Students were asked to feel the touch of the air inside the nostrils and imagine it travelling right down to the pelvic region, through the different types of pranayamic techniques.

Imparting Instructions in Kriyas

Techniques of Kapalbhati (exhaling rapidly using forceful abdominal movements), Uddiyana (exhaling fully, pull back the abdominal muscles and lift upwards against the diaphragm, holding with breath out for a few seconds), and Agnisara (flapping tummy muscles in and out) were explained to the class, and they were asked to appreciate the influence of these techniques on the internal feeling of the touch of air.

'OM' recitation was given in a bass tone, with emphasis on starting the recitation below the umbilicus and slowly taking it up to the forehead. Gradually the vibratory aspect of the 'OM' was introduced to the class, and they were asked to experience these vibrations all over the body while reciting 'OM' in a relaxed manner.

After four weeks of yoga practice, discussions took place with each participant. It was ascertained that they had all developed better and better experiential awareness of the physical body, of their breathing movements, and of the 'OM' vibrations, giving them an enjoyable inner experience. Thus, the period in which they remained in this state was increased from five to ten minutes in the sixth week.

Yoga techniques like asanas, pranayamas, kriyas, and the 'OM' recitation were taught for 1½ hours every day for five days a week. It was realised that this method of teaching was close to the yogic line of thinking, where the student is expected to gain awareness of the interior of the body without using the sensory or motor organs (pratyahara).

At the end of the course, further tests and discussions took place with the participants. It was evident that physically handicapped people like the blind could be led to take an interest in themselves and their own welfare with positive motivation. They began to experience positive joy through the yoga techniques provided; these were given in a judicious and intelligent way.

After 1½ and 4½ months, follow-up studies were carried out by repeating interviews with the people concerned. Any mistakes or difficulties were rectified by checking exercises and giving practical guidance. During the follow-up studies it was realised that the participants had to spend about 1½ hours daily in yogic training. This had reduced their working hours and resulted in financial loss for the home. As this had not been foreseen when the project was planned, this could not be compensated. Thus, a third follow-up study was dropped. However, it was clear that the participants had experienced great benefit in the shape of a feeling of wellbeing, greater confidence to cope with their disabilities, improvement in behaviour and a developing interest in life and living. It is suggested that the financial loss incurred by the home should be taken into account for planning any such project in the future.

Dr Salam said, 'As soon as the programme is approved by the Government, we may be in a position to select a set of instructors working with other handicapped people, to go to Kaivalyadhama and train for one month in a systematised form of yoga teaching so that they can teach yoga exercises to small groups of the physically handicapped. The teachers would have just enough basic knowledge and experience of yoga not to get bogged down with technique and theory.'

Visit to the NAB Lions Home for the Aging Blind

We were welcomed to the NAB Lions Home by the Supervisor, Mr S.S. Pradhan. The Home was brightly decorated with Christmas paper chains, and the Superintendent, Mr Joshi, told us that Christmas was celebrated in the Home for the inmates' enjoyment, even though it was not a Hindu festival. The Home was set in beautiful gardens, surrounded by hills, and Mr Joshi said, 'We believe it's so important to have beautiful surroundings, because, even though the patients cannot see, they are still benefited by the atmosphere and peace.'

Mr Joshi had worked in his profession, dealing mainly with physically handicapped people, for 45 years. The Home housed up to 95 male inmates, aged 55 or over, looked after by 24 staff. Every applicant was fully assessed before admission. This was to ascertain temperament and make sure he would fit in with the others. The Home was financed by donations received mainly from

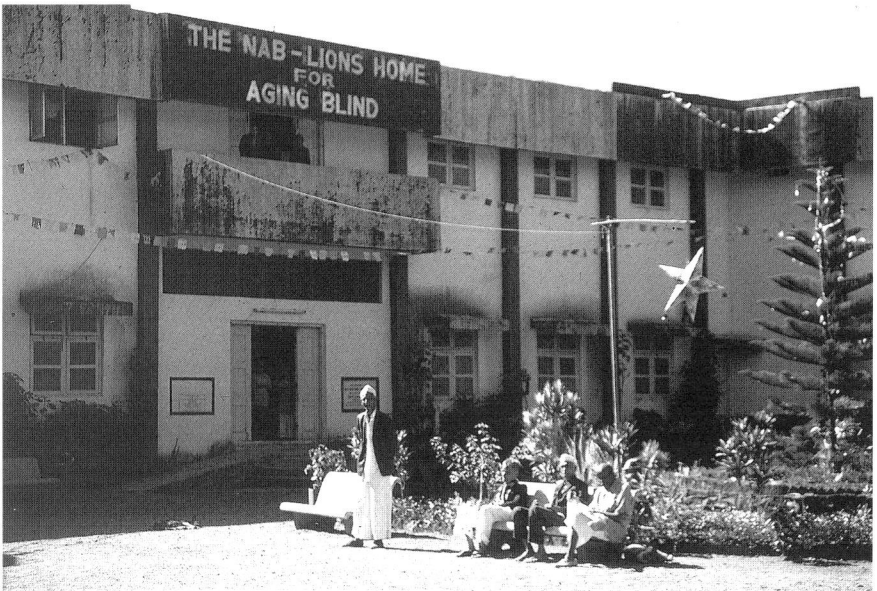

The Aging Blind Home, Khandala.

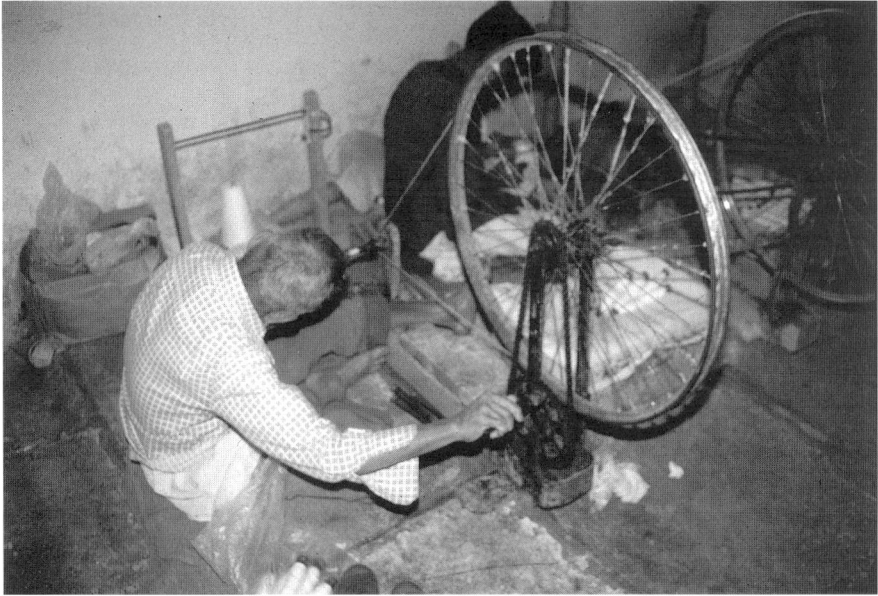

An inmate spinning on a loom.

the Lions organisation and from West Germany. Residence was free to the inmates, who were all blind or partially sighted. They were able to spin on looms, and to make candles, chalk and cardboard boxes. They were paid for this work which was mostly sold in Bombay. 'So the Home is not a dead end for them,' said Mr Joshi, 'they have something worthwhile to do, and they have a sense of independence.'

Mr A.N.V. Subramainiam Iyer, the librarian and braille teacher, who was himself blind, showed us several braille magazines received from the United Kingdom and the United States. He asked one inmate, who at the age of fifty-four had mastered English braille, Grade 1, within a month, to give a demonstration of dictation for overseas correspondence. We watched this gentleman write in braille: 'We thank you for sending the latest braille edition of the Oxford English Dictionary in the English language.'

The Supervisor took us round the Home and showed us the dormitories, the dining-room which seated a hundred people, and the various workshop rooms. There the inmates worked from 8 a.m. till noon, and then, after a two-hour gap for lunch and rest, carried on till 5 p.m.

The yoga practice took place at 6 a.m. each morning. During our visit, some of the inmates gave us a demonstration conducted by a female member of staff who had learnt the practice from the visiting yoga instructors from Kaivalyadhama during the three-month training programme. The inmates performed breathing exercises, leg-lifts, stretching (in Tadasana), Knee to Head Pose (Pashimottasana), Locust Posture (Salabhasana) and a vigorous backbending movement. At the end of the demonstration the Supervisor asked what they thought of their yoga practice, most of them replying that the effects were good and they felt refreshed. So even at this comparatively late stage in life, it is still a good time to do yoga!

Addresses:
Dr F.S. Abdul. Salam, Directorate of Social Welfare – Maharashtra State, 3 Church Road, PUNE – 411 001

Nab-Lions Home for Aging Blind, Sudder Baug, Old Khandala Road, KHANDALA, Bombay – 410 302

CHAPTER SIX

Meeting the Vora family – a meeting which opened many new and exciting doors for me

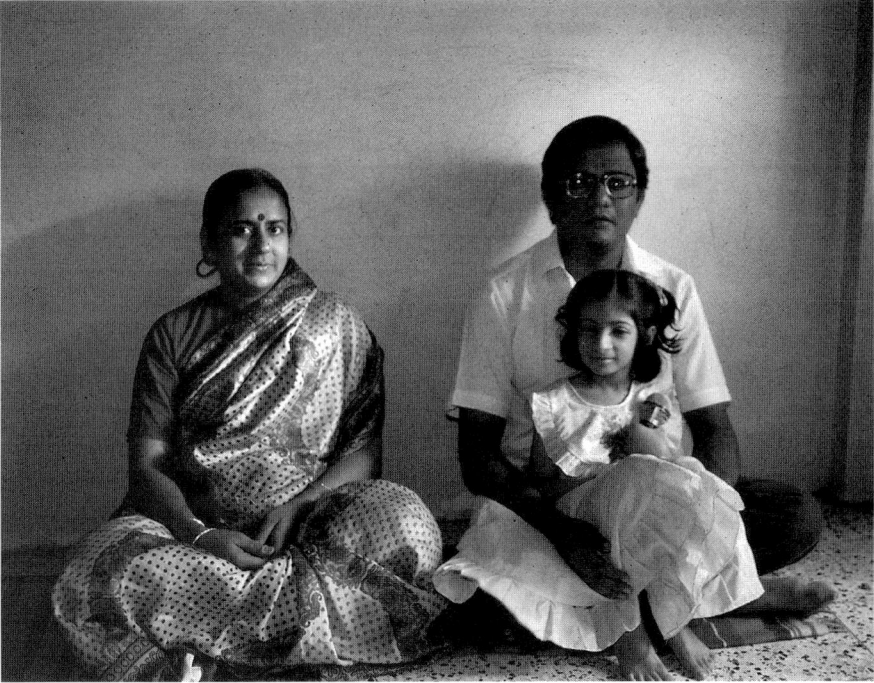

Mr and Mrs Vora and Tejal.

Some of the following was published in the *YOGA and Health Journal*, March 1990.

Mr Vora introduced himself to me after my talk and video given at the Yoga and Research Conference at Kaivalyadhama on 'Yoga for People with Learning Difficulties'. He told me that he had a daughter with Down's syndrome – Tejal, aged seven – and said how much he would like to have yoga taught in her special school.

It transpired that he had first come in contact with yoga 1½ years earlier through a friend who was having regular yoga therapy. Mr Vora and his friend met at 5 a.m. most mornings to attend various yoga sessions all over Bombay, and his friend's health had improved in consequence. Mr Vora had his own business in rubber and plastic raw materials and chemicals, and he invited Chris and myself to visit his home in Bombay and meet his family. We accepted gladly.

Mr Vora's home was a third-floor flat with two rooms, kitchen and bathroom. It was shared with his brother's family, including two children. As Tejal had an older brother, there were four children altogether. At home the family spoke Gujarati.

Tejal was accepted by all the children as an equal, although her speech was underdeveloped and her reactions slow. When she was four months old, her parents had noticed a deformity in both legs, and had taken her to the Rehabilitation Centre where plaster casts were placed on her legs. These were removed some time later. Fortunately her legs had straightened. She had begun to walk at the age of five and could now walk quite normally.

Tejal's parents had taken her to various medical and educational authorities in Bombay to make sure that she got the right schooling for her capabilities. She was now at Kalyandeep School, where she was given special education, and her parents and aunt continued to educate her at home to the best of their ability. Her mother took her to school every day. As the school was an hour's journey from the home, this meant a total of four hours travelling for the mother, who at that time was five months pregnant. She did it gladly however, for she and her husband could not do enough for the little girl. Mr Vora said of her, 'The Lord has given me this lovely child, whom I regard as a symbol of love in my home. Let us prove that it is a symbol of love in society also.'

Tejal, having played freely at home with the other children, found it easy to mix with her fellow pupils, and was relaxed and confident. She was obedient, polite, and very affectionate – a most lovable child. It was encouraging that she enjoyed watching television, with no difficulty in concentrating.

Tejal's aunt had attended a short yoga course at The Yoga Institute in Santa Cruz and practised at home. Tejal had learnt some of the exercises from her aunt and the two of them gave us a joint demonstration. Tejal copied some postures I showed her and had no apparent difficulty in following my English instructions. We were told that her concentration had improved considerably since she started yoga and I suggested that Mr Vora should take her to a private yoga teacher.

Mr and Mrs Vora entertained us to a splendid Jain meal. They made a point of including Tejal in the conversation and she responded well. Mr Vora then suggested that we should accompany him and his wife to an appointment they had with Tejal's psychologist/counsellor at the clinic. This lady, Miss D'Silva, was pleased to see us and asked me about my work. She then told me something about her own work with Tejal, in which she used psychological testing techniques and scientific testing equipment. She also gave counselling to the parents with a team of health and education experts from social services. Miss D'Silva stressed the importance of workers for the disabled fully cooperating with each other and sharing problems and experiences to mutual benefit. In addition to us visiting Tejal's school, Kalyandeep, Miss D'Silva recommended that we visit her at Dilkhush Special School where yoga took place every other day for some of the children.

We were grateful to Mr and Mrs Vora for giving up their appointment with Miss D'Silva so that we could talk with her ourselves. In fact, Mr Vora's enthusiasm for his daughter's welfare and his desire to assist me in my Fellowship investigations resulted in invaluable further contacts.

CHAPTER SEVEN

Our Visit to Dilkhush Special School

The word 'Dil' means heart, and 'Khush' means happy, so Dilkhush means 'The Happy Heart' – a most appropriate name.

In 1970 it was estimated that 3 per cent of the population had learning difficulties and/or disabilities. At that time there was only one institution in Bombay, training a few teachers in special education, for such people.

In 1971 the Handmaids of the sacred Heart of the Society of Jesus started Dilkhush Special School at Juhu. Five of the Sisters had trained in Special Education at the world-famous Institutions of St Michael and St John in Dublin, and another teacher assisted them when the school started with fifteen pupils. The Sisters, realising that it was essential to have a sufficient number of trained teachers, also established the Dilkhush Teachers' Training Centre, a Government-recognised centre which trained twelve teachers each year in methods of educating disabled children. In 1975 an extra building was built for the Dilkhush Vocational Centre. Here pupils were trained for work once they had finished their schooling.

When we visited Dilkhush in January 1985, there were 119 pupils. A number of the poorer ones received their education free or paid a mere concessionary fee. The school consisted of a spacious building, a well laid out garden and play areas with slides, swings and see-saws. At that time, there were six sisters, eight teachers, a P.T. master, a yoga teacher, an Indian music master, a paediatrician, a speech therapist and a psychologist. The Dilkhush complex was closely bonded together by cooperation between the Sisters, the staff and the parents. This cooperation between dedicated groups ensured that, even though the disabled children might be the victims of fate, they would certainly not be the victims of neglect.

The schooling at Dilkhush taught the children self-expression and self-care, aiming to make them useful members of society. Unlike ordinary schools, it catered for all children with a slow-learning ability. The children were grouped as follows: kindergarten, pre-school, junior, transition, intermediate and senior. There were also groups of activity classes, one being occupational home science which included cooking, stitching and housework. The senior group concentrated on pre-vocational classes, working with their hands to prepare for future work in the sheltered workshop. Here they worked with machinery and various materials to produce gift articles, handicrafts in wood, teaching aids, greeting cards, envelopes and small plaster statues. In this group there was one teacher to every ten or twelve children.

The Principal, Sister Maria Dolores Tena, said that she reckoned they had as many teaching methods as they had children! Methods used included Montessori and others, but the best method of all she said, was love. This, coupled with understanding, bore out the school's excellent motto. 'Accept me as I am, only then will we discover each other.'

The Teachers' Training Course was a full-time course lasting a year and was confined to applicants who were considered to be temperamentally suited to this special type of teaching. On completion, the teachers received a diploma or a certificate in Special Education according to the examination marks they obtained.

With regard to practical classwork training, Sister Dolores said that the teacher trainees helped the teachers and gave individual tuition to the children. Miss Moffit, who had been a teacher at Dilkhush since 1973, explained that each month they had one of the trainee teachers along to attend in a classroom. For the first week, the trainee spent observing the children's responses to the teacher's instructions. Subsequently, the teacher instructed the trainee in what to do and towards the end of the month the trainee was competent to be left on her own with the children. One of the trainees told me that after studying the theory, the practical experience in the class room under the teacher's guidance gave her valuable insights into the various methods of dealing with children. 'These children are special, so we can't just experiment with them.'

Sister Dolores said that considerable time was spent working with parents, who seemed to need at least as much guidance as the children. Dilkhush had an active Parent Teacher Association and through meetings the school was able to give both parents and the whole family help in bringing up and understanding the needs of their children. Because the children loved the teachers, the parents loved them too. The parents were asked to fill in a questionnaire; and if there were any special difficulties Sister Dolores and Miss D'Silva, the psychologist, visited the family to discuss and deal with the problems. It was impressed upon the parents that they must first accept the child 'as I am'. Only then could advice be given as to how to handle the child in the context of the family. The whole arrangement worked very well.

Sister Dolores took us to see the class activities. The kindergarten class were outside in the garden doing their daily exercises, which began with running, followed by forward bends, backward bends, raising their arms, turning their hands around, and finished with attempts to jump (not all of them successful). These exercises benefited the children's physical coordination.

At lunchtime the kindergarten, preschool and junior groups were helped with their food by the teachers and some of the older Occupational Home Science pupils. The intermediate class, consisting of five girls and six boys, had just finished a language lesson and were writing it up in their workbooks. The senior class had varying levels of ability in reading and maths, and they were taught general knowledge and given plenty of map work. Their mental age was 6 to 10, although their actual ages ranged from 13 to 20.

Sister Esperença Martin was Director of the Vocational Centre where there were fourteen boys and four girls making educational wooden toys. These were finished so well that orders were received

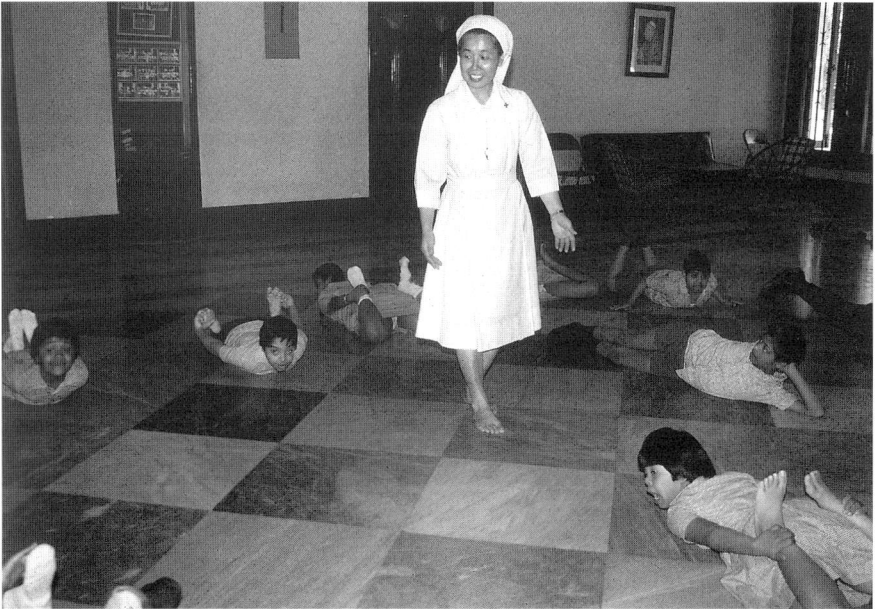

Sister Asunta Nakade giving her junior class a yoga lesson.

from Japan, America and other countries, as well as schools in Bombay. In fact, seven of the children had become so expert that they could earn up to 250 rupees a week, a good wage for a worker in Bombay.

In the main assembly hall Sister Asunta Nakade was giving her junior class a 20-minute yoga lesson. Five years earlier she had done a month's yoga training at The Yoga Institute in Santa Cruz and since then she had been giving yoga lessons to her group three times a week. She first gave a demonstration and then the children imitated her movements. She maintained their attention by blowing a whistle every time she changed posture.

The procedure of the yoga session was as follows:

1. Sitting in Namaste with hands in the prayer position

2. Sitting in Padmasana (the lotus position) with eyes closed

3. Yogamudra – from Padmasana, bending forward and down towards each knee in turn

4. Ishwana Pranamudra – arms raised in prayer (the 'surrender to God' gesture)

5. Pashimottasana – legs stretched forward while bending head forward and down

6. Dhanarasana – roll on to front and clasp hands around feet in the Bow position

7. Hugging knees in crouched position

The perfect control exhibited by this group filled us with admiration.

Our visit was rounded off by all the children gathering together and giving us a musical show of nursery rhymes accompanied on the piano, followed by their acting out the dramas of Little Bo Peep, Little Jack Horner, and Jack and Jill.

The children appeared very happy at Dilkhush and it was clear that they had benefited greatly from their Special Education. To most of them attending school was a treat, having to stay away was a punishment.

Miss D'Silva, Psychologist, commented after the guided tour

'Yoga is a very fine field for our disabled children, because it is a special channel through which we can vitalise the body, mind, soul and heart. I feel heartened by the children at Dilkhush who have been practising yoga under Sister Asunta Nakade's training.

She is Japanese, and as you know, the Japanese are well-known for their precision. The way she does yoga with the children is wonderful, and has given me hope that they may be able to use their minds and bodies profitably throughout their lives.

'I have been the psychologist at Dilkhush from the time the school started in 1971. I have done my Master of Education and specialist training in Special Needs. Besides visiting Dilkhush, I go to various other institutes for disabled children, to an ordinary High School and its Special Education Department, and to a special Gujarati School. I have also started a small private training programme for children with learning disabilities and I have two private clinics.

'In my private clinics I only take three children a day. I give them 45 to 50 minute appointments, because I think these children need a lot of help, and if I were to work only 15-minute sessions with them, I would not be doing them justice, and would be thinking about the next appointment.'

Miss D'Silva went on to describe her counselling work with the parents of her disabled pupils. She said that in general the parents were anxious to help their children to lead normal lives, but there were some who did not really accept the child. This was because they were conditioned by the Indian philosophy according to which a disabled child is the result of bad karma (the operation of the law of cause and effect working out from one life to another). Having such a child reflected on them, which made them reluctant to exhibit the child in society. In some extreme cases, handicap was regarded as a disease and the child was considered an untouchable. Parents of normal children might go so far as to keep their child away from the disabled one, in case their child might contract a similar disability.

All these problems had to be overcome by Miss D'Silva emphasising that God loves the disabled child just as he or she is and this had to be accepted not only by the parents, but by all other members of the family. This is because when an Indian girl marries she becomes related to her husband's entire family and they must all be persuaded to accept the new liberal viewpoint. Eventually the child would be recognised by society as a valuable member of the community, particularly when he or she was able to work and earn a little money at the age of 16–20. Miss D'Silva said she found this aspect of her work very rewarding.

Address:
Dilkhush Special School, Church Road, JUHU, Bombay – 400 049.

CHAPTER EIGHT

A Visit to Kalyandeep Special School (Tejal's School)

In 1955 Bhagini Seva Mandir Kumarika Stree Mandel founded this school with three children with learning difficulties. The school was renamed Kalyandeep Special School in 1980 as a result of a generous donation for the extension of the school building by Shri Vivendrabhai Nanavaty in memory of his late father. The word 'kalyan' means welfare, and 'deep' means light. The school is recognised by the Directorate of Social Welfare, Maharashtra State.

Kalyandeep's objectives are as follows:

- To make society aware of the needs of the children through various integrated programmes

- To allow children to develop in a free and fearless atmosphere to their fullest capacity

- To train them in self-care

- To give them pre-vocational and vocational training

- To find them work in suitable industries outside

- To give work to disabled adults who cannot be absorbed into the open market.

Tejal's teacher, Ms P.A. Mehta, took us round the various classrooms, which consisted of a preparatory class for very young children and their families, a primary class, a junior class, an intermediate class and a senior class.

In addition to training the children in routine daily living, they were given pre-vocational training in making chalk, together with boxes, which were supplied to schools and colleges in Bombay. They were also taught screen printing, bookbinding, sewing and embroidery and made blackboard dusters, paper bags for groceries, office envelopes, fancy envelopes and greeting cards.

Ms Mehta told me that when Tejal started the school she spoke very little, but her speech was now much improved. Previously she had been hyperactive, and she kept getting up restlessly and wandering around, but she was now relaxed and she had begun to take an interest in all the lessons and class activities.

We were next introduced to Mrs Latha Katarine, the Honorary Director of the School. She told us that in addition to the special teaching given in the classrooms, there were members of para-medical staff such as speech therapists, occupational therapists and psychotherapists who trained and educated the children. All the teachers kept in close touch with parents through meetings and home visits. Attached to the Special School there was also a Primary Teachers' Training College, and a Primary Mainstream School. As all the children were on the same premises, Kalyandeep based its approach on integration wherever there was some form of collective activity involved. For instance, the children were combined in sports, trips and cultural activities. Within four years the integration programme had enabled five children from the special school aged between five and eight to be absorbed into the mainstream school. Three disabled adults had been placed in outside jobs, and their employers' reports on their work had been excellent.

I was so pleased when Mrs Katarine told me that the pupils aged between ten and twenty were also taught yoga. She said, 'Our yoga teacher comes every week for two hours to teach them to meditate, concentrate, and do various postures. He teaches the postures with the mantra 'OM SHANTI', which assists concen-tration, so that restless children can concentrate better and do a particular activity for a slightly longer period. As a result they feel happy and content, and we have found definite improvement through the yoga.'

Mr Vora must have been surprised and pleased to learn that after all Tejal would be receiving yoga education at school as soon as she reached the age of ten.

As we were leaving, Ms Mehta said that she would ask the yoga teacher if he could start yoga with her class. She showed me the book they used at the school called 'Teaching Yogasana to the Mentally Retarded' by Dr Jeyachandran of the Vijay Human Services in Madras.

To my surprise and delight I learned from this book that the techniques which were being used for the children were the same techniques that I had found suitable for the adults with learning difficulties while working at ILEA for the past six years – a true meeting of minds! I set out to meet this man who had initiated the teaching of yoga at the school, Dr Jeyachandran, Director of Special Education for Children and Teacher Training Programmes in Madras.

Address:
Kalyandeep Special School, Sarojin Road, VILE-PARLE (West), Bombay, 400 056,

CHAPTER NINE

The Highlight of my Fellowship – Meeting Dr P. Jeyachandran

In January 1985, after several thousands of miles of travel, I eventually met Dr Jeyachandran in Madras at Vijay Human Services – a small school for children with learning difficulties. He greeted me with surprise to learn that even though we were at opposite ends of the earth, we had both introduced yoga to people with severe learning difficulties at around the same time. I told him that I had been working along similar lines to his, with regard to the techniques training of staff working in special needs. He was truly amazed at the coincidence. This confirmed my confidence in my own beliefs and work.

Dr Jeyachandran told me about the facilities at his training schools where he is the Director of Special Education for Children

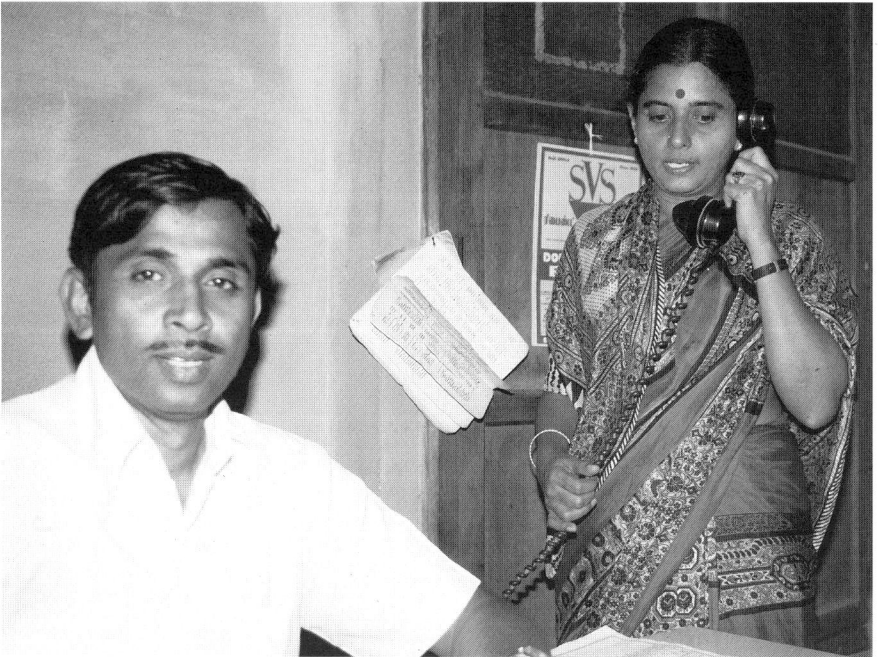

Dr P. Jeyachandran, Director of Special Education, Tamil Nadu, and Ms Vimla, Principal, Bala Vihar Training School.

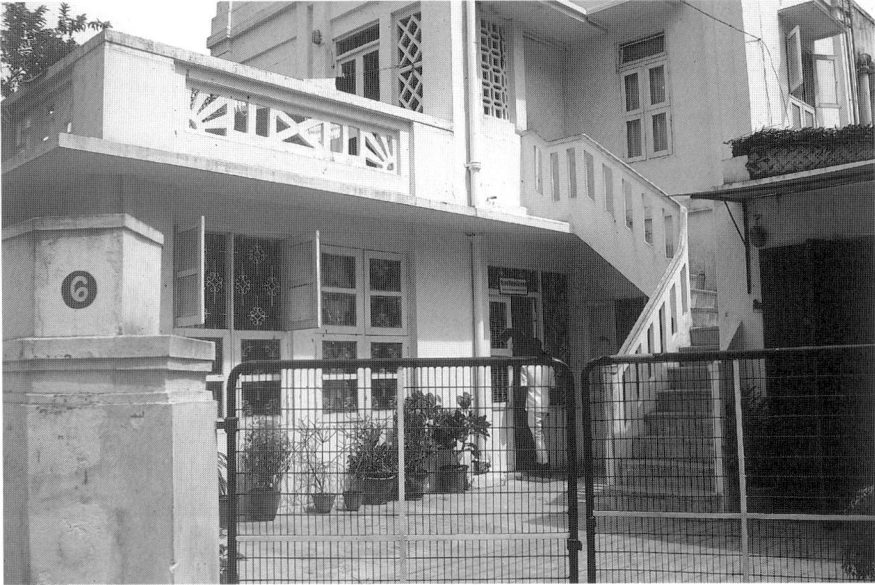

The Headquarters of Vijay Human Services.

and the Teacher-Training Programmes in Madras. He became Director of Balar Vihar Special Education Training Centres following his Master's degree in Psychology and research into disability, and his research programmes on training the parents of disabled children.

Dr Jeyachandran found he did not have the necessary freedom to deal with the special needs of some of the children with severe learning disabilities, so he initiated Vijay Human Services. This was a registered organisation which provided schooling for those disabled children who had been rejected by all other institutions for the disabled – this being the criterion for admission. Jeyachandran had two other psychologists to assist him – Ms Lata Kumar, Principal of Vijay Human Services and Ms Vimla, Principal of Bala Vihar Training School.

He showed me the 1985 Special Education curriculum for training special educators and parents to teach yoga to children with severe learning difficulties. Dr Jeyachandran, and his two other assistant psychologists, had devised a yoga programme for children with learning difficulties which was included in the syllabus. Their ten years of research showed that such children could be greatly helped by a series of fourteen yogasanas (postures) which were simple to learn and did not require much effort, accompanied by the utterance of various sounds which enabled the children to exhale in rhythm with the movements. Relaxation periods were also a planned part of the programme.

In India, since the early eighties, yoga has been a part of the Special Education system and children with severe learning difficulties have been successfully practising basic techniques in yoga, breathing and relaxation. Dr Jeyachandran and his interdisciplinary team have studied the effects of yoga on the children, their parents/guardians and special educators, and concluded that the regular practise of yoga benefits both pupils and practitioners. The team consider that the yoga syllabus complements the conventional-behaviour-modification special schooling system which they have adopted from the west.

Their work was based on the following three projects:

1. The methods of teaching yogasana to children with learning difficulties.
2. Madras Developmental Programming System's Behaviour Scales.
3. A national teacher-training curriculum in Special Education.

Project One.
The methods of teaching yogasana to the children

In the trial project in 1982, Jeyachandran was assisted by Krishnamacharya Yoga Mandiram and about ten other agencies. A yoga teacher originally visited the school to teach yoga to the children and the special educators assisted her. She found that the special educators with the most experience in handling disabled children were able to get the best out of them when teaching them yoga.

They next investigated the training of special educators for the children. When describing their work to me Dr Jeyachandran said, 'You won't believe this, but the results were the greatest surprise I have ever had. Each one of the teacher trainees came to me and said in effect, 'I had a health problem, but since practising the yoga I have been better'. The ailments which improved included giddiness, irregular menstruation, headaches, asthma, and spondylitis.'

Although the programme succeeded in improving adaptive behaviour, a clear and comprehensive guide for those who lived and worked with the disabled child had never been devised. With this in mind, Jeyachandran went to see Krishnamacharya, who was in his late nineties and who was the original Guru to the famous B.K.S. Iyengar. Krishnamacharya much admired the work of Vijay Human Services, and agreed to advise on the teaching of yoga to the special educators, but asked for Jeyachandran's own suggestions as to what could be taught to the children with learning difficulties and disabilities. Krishnamacharya expressed great interest in the project and asked to be kept informed of progress.

Report on the Yoga Study Programme

This report is by the Krishnamacharya Yoga Mandiram (a yoga therapeutic centre registered with the Health Ministry) in collaboration with Vijay Human Services

The study was on yoga for children with severe learning difficulties. The aim was to train special educators to teach such pupils to practise asanas (postures) and pranayama (breathing practices).

Subjects

Fifty children and twenty-one special educators were chosen to participate in the project. The children were drawn from three centres located in Madras and were selected on the basis of age, I.Q., and absence of serious hearing or visual problems. There were thirty-six boys and fourteen girls ranging in age from eight to sixteen, though most of them were twelve.

All the special educators and trainees who took part had a teacher-training qualification and at least three months' experience in handling disabled children.

The course

The educators were given one-hour sessions a week in asana and pranayama lessons over a period of twelve weeks. Following the first two weeks they were instructed to teach the children for half-an-hour a day on six days a week for the remainder of the course.

To start with, Jeyachandran introduced the educators to their yoga teacher from Krishnamacharya Yoga Mandiram, who showed them diagrams of the asanas (postures) and pranayama (breathing) practices to be used in their own course in one-hour sessions. They were asked, while practising yoga on their own for thirty minutes a day, to consider the methods they would use to teach the children. The third week each of them was deputed to teach the same yogasana (yoga postures) for half-an-hour to two or three children. In this way, they gained knowledge and experience of yoga, so that the complicated problems they encountered during the teaching could be referred to the yoga teacher for elucidation. In addition, other members of the teaching staff advised them how to handle general problems.

The educators gained benefit from their own practice. The change they could see in their own physical well-being increased their confidence and encouraged them to look for similar results in the children.

Assessment of Children's Progress

Assessment was done on the basis of observations and case studies by the special educators who checked with the parents, residential staff and course organisers. The improvements in the fifty children were as follows: reduced drooling and obesity; disappearance of facial tics, thumb-sucking and wheezing; improvement in posture while standing or walking; improvement in appetite and sleeping; improvement in gross and fine motor skills; improved behaviour; reduction in hyperactivity; improved speech and a new ability to interact socially.

By the end of the yoga study programme Jeyachandran was able to report to Krishnamacharya that the children had achieved an encouraging degree of proficiency in yoga, and the confidence this engendered helped them to learn new skills and to participate more efficiently in practice. Also their behaviour showed improvement not only in the motor training areas as expected, but in other areas as well such as: eating, dressing, behaviour, social interaction and language development.

Observations by Educators

The benefits the educators experienced were: reduced tension; diminished abdomen size; improved appetite; elimination of drugs for painful or irregular periods; fewer headaches; improved sleeping; control of such problems as irritable colon and peptic ulcer; control of diabetes without medication; relief of knee pain and swelling in the legs; relief of giddiness and blackouts; alleviation of the discomforts of pregnancy.

All these benefits to both pupils and educators occurred simply through the basic course, with no special yoga treatment for specific problems

The educators have continued teaching in different parts of India, and have kept Dr Jeyachandran informed of the progress their pupils have made, which he found very encouraging.

Contributions made by Desikachar

It was fortunate that Desikachar, the son of Krishnamacharya, was able to assist Jeyachandran with the project, giving insight and confidence to the educators. Desikachar emphasised to me in our meeting how dedicated Jeyachandran had been to all his work for disabled children. He said the work involved three processes:

1. The specific yoga teachers' training programme
2. The special needs of the disabled child (dealt with in the Madras Developmental Behaviour Scales in next project)
3. Counselling with the child's family.

According to Desikachar, planning for the practice of yogasana is of great importance, especially when devising individualised programmes plans. The first step is to discover the pupil's 'starting-point' according to their capabilities, by seeing whether they are able to stand, bend, sit up, lie down and then stand up, and move both sides of the body. The simplest movements are generally raising the arms, bending forward, lying down, and lifting each leg in turn. The aim is to loosen-up the joints gradually in order to transfer energy to that part of the body which needs to be stimulated.

Planning for the practice of yogasana is worked out through the process of 'Vinyasa'. Vinyasa means devising an organised sequence of asanas planned with discrimination to suit the needs and abilities of the pupil and lead to the desired goal. Vinyasa applies not only to a sequence of asanas, but also to a single asana, so that the pupil can progress gradually from a dynamic to a static posture. Practising dynamically is through repetition. Practising statically is through holding the posture.

A 'main posture' is chosen to meet individual needs and abilities. Before starting a posture, you must ensure that you know the appropriate warming-up movements enabling you to build up to the main posture, and the counterpostures enabling you to descend and unwind comfortably back to a relaxed position.

Desikachar said, 'It was the aim of special education yoga teachers to encourage the children's parents to practise with their children at home, thus reinforcing the lessons learned at school. The parents and the residential staff were encouraged to join in the lessons, and asked to report back any problems, achievements etc. which could then be discussed with the teachers.

'Yoga has given these children more interest and has improved their self-esteem and their attitude to their families and outsiders.' Desikachar was amazed and delighted that new programmes were still instituted every week and also that the enthusiasm of the special educators was constantly maintained. He said there was no doubt that the yoga programme was helpful to the disabled children, particularly in view of a change of attitude from regarding the children almost as inanimate objects, to treating them as persons in their own right who could be active participants in their own development. Although at that time he had little knowledge of children with learning difficulties and/or disabilities, he had always taught that yoga can be adapted to fit the needs of any individual and this led him to study the special requirements of these children and understand how asanas could provide some hope for their improvement in both behaviour and general attitude. His book 'Religiousness in Yoga: Lectures on Theory and Practice' was helpful in defining the meaning of yoga in special education. He also helped the course organisers to select suitable asanas, pranayamas and relaxation techniques for the children, together with the teaching strategies to be used.

Project Two.
Madras Developmental Programming System

All the children who attend Balar Vilar Special Education schools have an individualised programme plan worked out according to the Madras Developmental Behaviour Scales. These are designed to provide information about the functional skills of the children with learning difficulties. The scales contain 360 items grouped under 18 functional sections, by means of which the educator assesses the child's behaviour and marks 'A' for what s/he can do, and 'B' for what s/he cannot do. This is a representation of the child's Behaviour Profile from which the interdisciplinary team decide upon the priority goals set for him during the next three months. Once the goals have been set, the education procedure is written up on the Individualised Programme Plan Form. This sets out the behaviour objectives required of the child, the conditions necessary to improve his behaviour, the strategic teaching methods to be used in accomplishing the goals and the name of the member of staff who has been deputed to teach him. Each special educator is assigned three to five pupils. Keeping records of the children's level of performance helps the interdisciplinary team to evaluate the percentage of each child's success rate by the date fixed for the quarterly Programme Plan. If they have accomplished the tasks, the next set of goals are planned for another three months' programme. If they have not, the same training must be gone through again.

Project Three.
A National Teacher-Training Curriculum for
Special Education

Dr Jeyachandran of the Bala Vihar school was chosen to compile the curriculum, assisted by an expert committee appointed by the Government of Tamil Nadu in South India. The work was finally completed in January 1985, at the time of our visit.

As cost was a major consideration, the organisers of the project were anxious to balance the cost against the need to train as many educators as possible without reducing the quality of the course. The conventional methods used were imported from the west, where a team of interdisciplinary workers combine in order to treat a single disabled child. However, this method of working is very expensive in both time and manpower, and has not always met the needs of the disabled in India. Consequently, it was decided that the Special Educators must assume the inherent responsibility for teaching the whole person. Special Educators would continue, however, to need the professional advice and assistance of medical and para-medical specialists. The training of the special educators is now designed to prepare them to implement and evaluate individualised programmes for the child. Plans are therefore based on the Individualised Programme Plan, which are jointly developed by the educators, parents, pupils and members of the interdisciplinary team.

Of course, the key to better service lies in staff training, for without capable staff even the most modern set-up can provide at best an indifferent service.

Course for Special Educators

This course of training is predominantly a professional and technical one, with eight examination subjects and six practical subjects which include teaching yoga techniques to improve general health, span of attention, motor coordination and social interaction of the child.

The special educators are taught that any disabled person, irrespective of the degree of handicap, is capable of learning something and that the responsibility for achieving the successive goals during the year lies with the educator rather than with the pupil. This way of looking at the learning process is a reversal of the usual one, where normally it is the pupil who must adapt to the educator's methods. If the pupil has failed to learn, the educator must ask in what respects did his/her lesson plan fail in its purpose, and s/he must then set about modifying the learning conditions accordingly. This form of educators' assessment is precisely how the basic principles of yoga practice are toned down and adjusted to suit the individual's need and capacity.

Jeyachandran concludes, 'A lot of work has been done to formulate our curriculum so as to include yoga and other ancient Indian teachings alongside contemporary western educational techniques. No complicated or highly specialised training has been necessary to enable Special Educators and parents to teach and practise with the children. The techniques can be readily passed on from one educator to another, so that this beneficial work is steadily growing.'

Dr Jeyachandran's special education programme in Madras exemplifies how yoga can become an integral part of the educational provision for the children's special needs. I am most grateful to him and his colleagues for being so open and willing to share their special work with me. My Churchill Report and Video on 'Yoga Therapy and Special Education in India' gives a full account of this research and curriculum. (Details given at end of this book.) Sir Richard Vickers, Director General, Churchill Trust has stated that this is 'a comprehensive and fascinating audio and visual report'.

The following publications provided some of my information and I would like to thank the authors and organisations responsible.

- *Teaching Yogasana to the Mentally Retarded* published by Krishnamacharya Mandiram in collaboration with Vijay Human Services, 1983, revised 1988.

- *A National Syllabus of Teacher Training for Special Education*, Dr Jeyachandran, Director, Balar Vihar Training School, Madras, 1985.

Addresses:

Vijay Human Services, 6 Lakshimipuram St, Rajapettah, MADRAS – 600 014.

Bala Vihar Training School, Kilpauk Gardens, MADRAS – 600 010.

Bahar Kalvi Nilayam, Balar Opportunity Section, Ritherdon Road, Vepery, MADRAS – 600 007.

CHAPTER TEN

Yoga for Aurally Impaired Children in conjunction with The Yoga Institute

A Pilot-Study Project Introduced by Ms Kalpana Shah

Following my correspondence with The Yoga Institute, Santa Cruz, Bombay, about Shri Yogendra's teachings, I was referred by the Principal, Dr Jayadeva, to Ms Kalpana Shah who had been teaching yoga to aurally impaired children. She spoke about her interest in the understanding of yoga. According to Kalpana Shah, with the passage of time one experiences an ever-growing need to live one's life more meaningfully. The study of yoga trains an individual in the understanding and appreciation of the various facets of our personalities: the body, mind, senses, intellect and character. We continually try to justify our actions on the ground of past experiences, personal satisfaction, even duty. Fulfilling one's duty towards humanity is universally considered noble and spiritual, but the performance of this duty must be supported by a spirit of dedication. Kalpana maintained, 'Serving disabled people must be seen as the sacred duty of each one of us'.

At the beginning of 1984, Dr Ajay Kothari, the Managing Trustee of Koshish School for Deaf Children, invited the authorities of the Yoga Institute to conduct yoga classes for the children, who totalled thirty, aged between four and twelve. Dr Kothari told us that the name of the school, Koshish, meant 'effort, which is what we encourage on the part of the teachers, parents, and children'. It appeared that 0.1 per cent of the Indian population was suffering from severe deafness. In Bombay, with a population of about nine million, there were approximately nine thousand severely deaf people (some of whom were also mute), with only eighteen schools for the deaf to cater for their needs. Koshish was perhaps the first private school in Bombay to provide free education and most of the children, who came from economically backward areas, were being educated free. Dr Kothari believed that every disabled child should be offered the same opportunities as normal children – this not only broadened horizons but could facilitate integration.

The training given included lip-reading, tactile vibrations and group-hearing-aid methods. Sign language was used only as a supplementary teaching method where necessary. Five teachers instructed these thirty children to communicate with speech and not with actions, sign language being practically banned. The Headteacher explained that auditory training with the use of earphones, hearing aids and lip-reading was the method of teaching the children, who had never heard normal children's babbling sounds such as ba-ba, da-da, and they did not know such sounds existed until they came to Koshish. Here the children were taught to speak as normally as possible, rather than communicate with sign-language alone. Initially the child was taught simply to make general vocal sounds. Next, they were taught how to pronounce particular sounds such as ah, pa, ba, ma, na, and after that words, followed by eventually speaking complete sentences.

Kalpana Shah, who trained as a yoga teacher at the Yoga Institute nine years previously, was responsible for the deaf children's yoga sessions, and during the initial stages was accompanied by another yoga teacher, Manahar Bhatia. Kalpana at first felt hesitant about imparting yoga teaching to these deaf and dumb children as she had only taught able-bodied pupils until then. It was through the guidance of Dr Jayadeva, Principal of the Yoga Institute, and through Kalpana's attendance at a few sessions at Koshish to learn some of their communication techniques, that she gained confidence for her new and challenging assignment.

Twenty-four, out of the thirty, children were allocated to the yoga sessions, which were held for one hour on four days each week. The first task of the two yoga teachers was to examine the case histories of the children. They found with most of them that complications had arisen due to illness, the taking of strong antibiotics by the mother during the last stages of pregnancy, or a forceps delivery.

During the first few sessions they had many problems. The school discouraged the use of sign language and stressed the need for lip-reading, thus communication at this stage presented many difficulties. It was essential to establish a good rapport with the children. Koshish School insisted that the children should try to speak to the yoga teachers and to each other as much as possible, and they made the wearing of hearing aids compulsory as this reduced the strain on the teachers. The yoga teachers employed the teaching methods of lip-reading and mirror-image action; for lip-reading the teacher must enunciate slowly, loudly and clearly for the children to follow what was being conveyed, while the mirror image action encouraged the children to imitate the teacher's movements.

Kalpana Shah described her experience at Koshish as one of the most demanding and fruitful teaching assignments of her career. In the course of this teaching she learned to be more humble, warm and compassionate – which she had never practised before coming into contact with these children. She discovered that what they needed in a world which too often turned its back on them and their handicap, was compassion, not pity. Compassion in the sense of recognising a need and having confidence in one's ability to meet it, rather than pity, focusing on and deploring a risk or disability. And they needed warmth, care and love. As a qualified yoga teacher, she was able to observe herself during the project, maintaining a good balance, being carried away by neither positive nor negative emotions. The satisfactory results she obtained with these deaf and dumb children convinced her that any handicap of language or limitation of communication could be overcome through the quality of love, which is the main pillar of the philosophy of yoga.

The Yoga Institute in Santa Cruz initially arranged for the aurally impaired children to have Hatha Yoga (physical training) only. After a few sessions these children easily performed the asanas, but the ability to breathe properly in asana still seemed to elude them. Yet coordinating breathing and body movements was essential for the successful practice of yoga. The children's school teachers requested Kalpana Shah concentrate on breathing techniques, because breathing plays a vital role in vibrations and speech. However, Kalpana Shah felt that these children would benefit more from a total yoga education programme. She therefore approached Dr Jayadeva, Principal of the Yoga Institute, and Dr Kothari at Koshish, for their advice and suggestions on how to organise a general yoga course for the four-month project. They willingly agreed to help, and the three of them prepared a syllabus together.

It was agreed that Kalpana should first focus on Pranayama (breath control) to enable the children to learn how to use different respiratory muscles and utilise to the full their breathing capacity, with the aim of helping their speech problem. Because of their hearing difficulties various strategies for teaching pranayama were devised:

1. For inhalation the children were made to concentrate on their throats and closely observe the slow and smooth passage of air.

2. For exhalation they were shown how to breathe out the air on to the backs of their arms, and to observe the sensation of warmth along with the movement of the tiny hairs on their arms, caused by the puff of air. Breathing out fully requires a conscious effort, and another technique used to emphasise exhalation was blowing into a balloon, which impressed on the children the effort needed to breathe out to the fullest extent. The direction of the exhaled breath was indicated by their blowing at the smoke from a burning incense stick.

3. The next stage was Pranayama One, the abdominal breathing technique where the diaphragm is forced to assist exhalation. The children picked this up quickly once they understood the breathing-out process.

4. Kapalabhati is the technique of making inhalation and exhalation follow each other in rapid succession without a break. To coordinate the breathing with sound, the children practised the rapid Kapalabhati technique while forcing out the sound 'OM' during each exhalation.

5. The yoga course included concentration and meditation exercises, the purpose of which was to help the children's mentality, since they were rather moody and their mental growth was slow. They were taught to concentrate and be still, so that while practising Pranayama they could increase the gap between exhalation and inhalation. The idea was that by increasing the space between each breath, they would be enabled to think faster. The hope was that through the yoga practices the children could be relieved of stress and frustration, and eventually attain a near-normal level of feeling, thinking and acting.

6. To help incorporate the benefit of asanas into the children's daily routine, they were taught to pick up objects from the floor without bending their knees. (I myself do not agree with this, which runs contrary to the western idea of always bending one's knees and keeping one's back straight when picking something up.) Another exercise the children particularly enjoyed was balancing on their toes while stretching their spines and reaching up to grasp something overhead.

The course was designed to instil in the child a sense of self-discipline so as to foster feelings of understanding, cooperation, and unity. This was done by doing simple things such as placing all their shoes neatly against the wall, standing in line, maintaining their own hearing aids, helping each other, being punctual, and observing personal hygiene and general cleanliness in the community.

Visit to a Yoga Session at Koshish

Dr Kothari and the teachers at the school welcomed us, and nine of the children assembled to take part. During the demonstration I was deeply impressed by the rapt attention the children gave to all Kalpana's movements and directions; and also by the near-unanimity with which they carried out her instructions. This clearly showed how successful she had been in her aim of forming a close and continuing bond and rapport with her disabled pupils, which is so essential if progress is to be made. I was fascinated by the methods Kalpana used to get through to the children and convey the essence of her yoga teaching to them, and I made videos of the procedure and took photographs, as shown here.

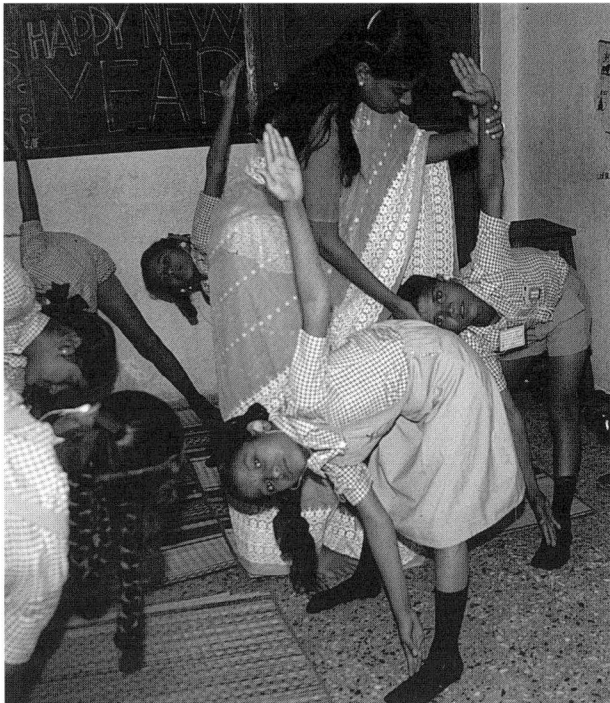

The children maintain balance while performing the Cross Triangle (Parivrtta Trikonasana).

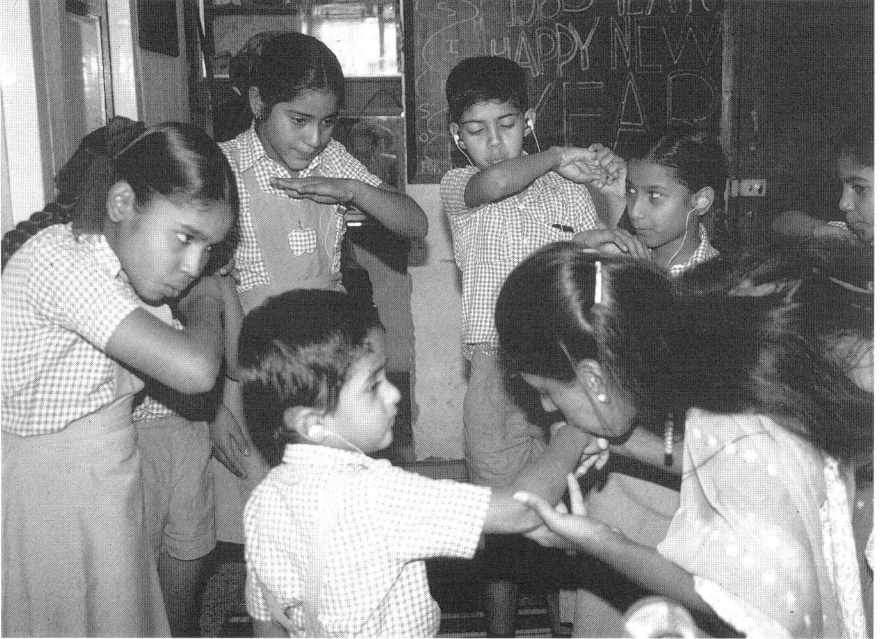

When exhaling, they were shown how to breathe out the air on to the backs of their arms.

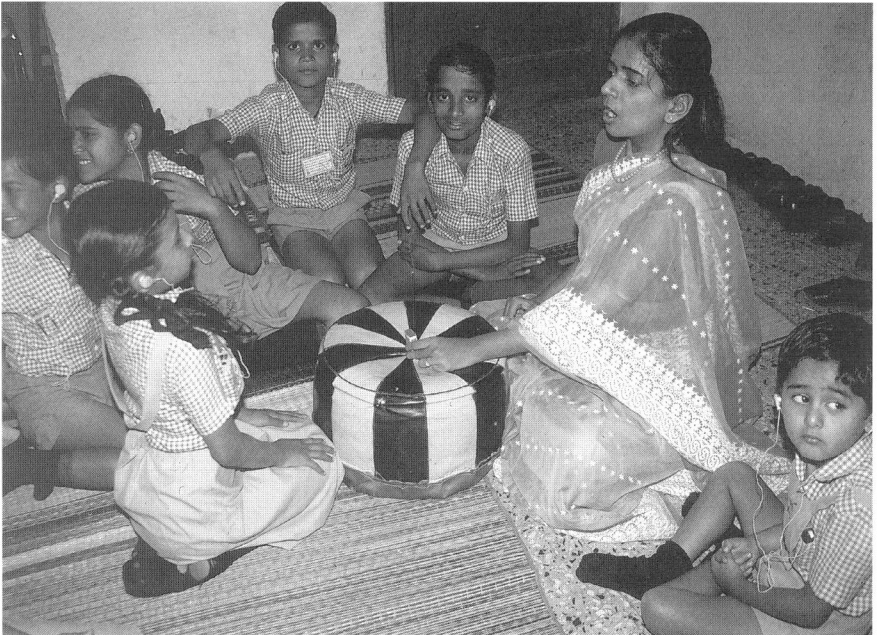

The direction of the children's exhaled breath was shown by their blowing at the smoke of a burning incense stick.

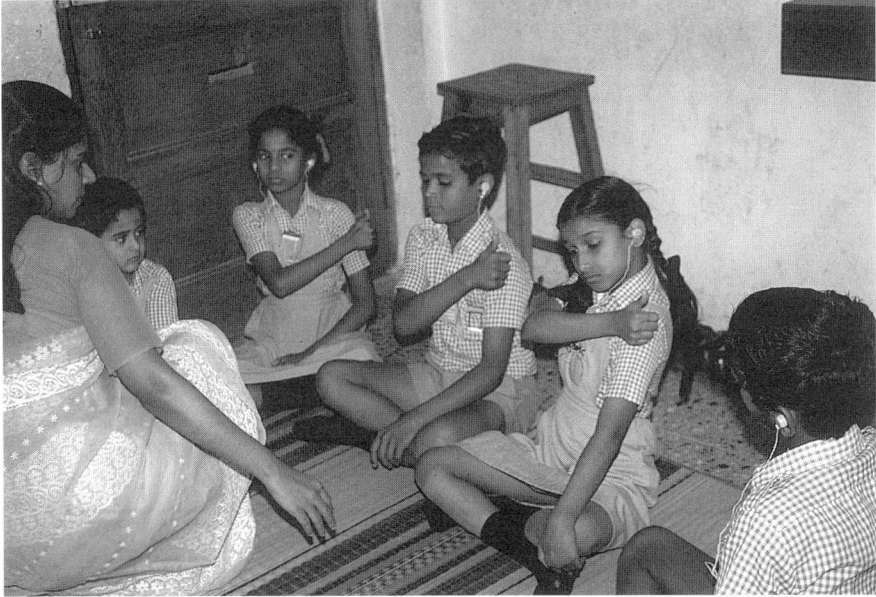

Following the thumb, an exercise for the eyes.

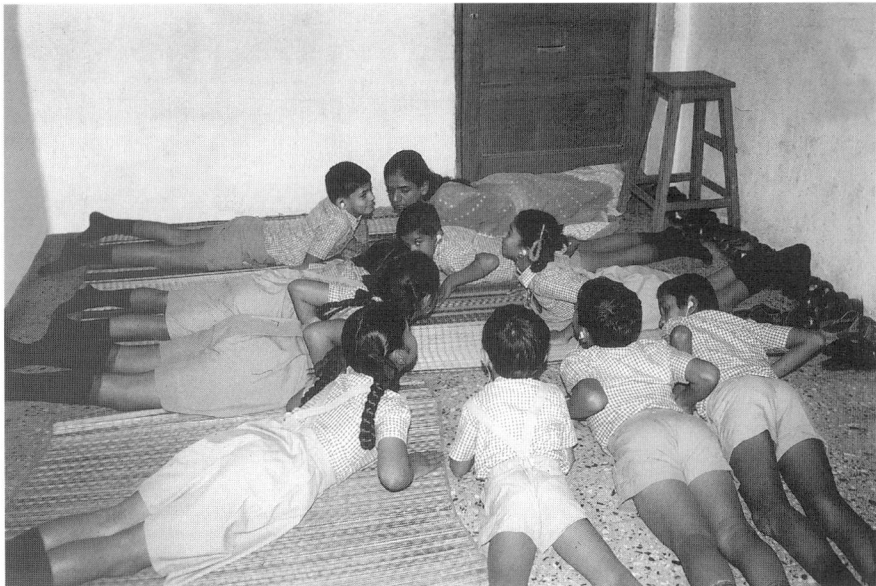

Kalpana and the children performing the Cobra pose (Bhujangasana).

I would like to mention how very warmly we were received by Kalpana's family who gave us wonderful hospitality.

CHAPTER TWELVE

Yoga with patients suffering from schizophrenia and various types of neurosis

Experiment with Yoga as a Therapy for Psychiatric Disorders, carried out at Psychiatric Department, Seth G.S. Medical College, and K.E.M. Hospital, Parel, Bombay.

Dr L. P. Shah, Professor of Psychiatry, stated, 'Psychiatric disorders pose challenging problems of management, and even after the introduction of modern techniques of therapy, limitations are not overcome'. Now that science has acknowledged that the mind has a direct influence on the body, some members of the medical profession are showing an interest in yoga therapy.

The clinical psychologist at the hospital suggested that yoga should be introduced, and this was agreed. A period of only four weeks was allocated to 'Study yoga as a treatment for anxiety neurosis', this project being financed by the Hospital Research Society. Clinical conditions were treated by drugs, psychotherapy, behaviour therapy, bio-feedback, and counselling. This report deals with the comparative evaluation of yoga therapy and behaviour therapy (i.e. deep muscle relaxation).

A number of patients were referred by the psychiatric outpatient department. They were seen by Dr Amresh Srivastava, the Research Officer, who gave them psychological tests. The Hamilton Anxiety and Depression Scales were administered to measure the degree of psychopathology. The diagnoses were confirmed by Professor Shah, the Consultant Psychiatrist, and detailed clinical data was collected.

The patients were then randomly divided into two groups, comprising thirty patients in each group. Placebo tablets (calcium lactate) were given to all of them. Group One received yoga therapy, and group two were given behaviour therapy.

Group One – The thirty patients received yoga therapy from Mrs Nilima Bhava, M.A., an experienced therapist assigned by Dr Jayadeva of the Yoga Institute. Before starting, she interviewed them all separately, collecting information about their personal and family backgrounds. She worked on the following basis:

According to yoga philosophy the mind functions on five levels:

1. Mudha – confused, agitated
2. Ksipta – distracted, unsteady
3. Viksipta – occasionally steady
4. Ekagra – one-pointed
5. Niruddha – controlled.

The first three categories denote a disturbed functioning of the mind, where awareness (objective thinking) is nil or very low.

Yoga discipline, both physical and mental, is intended gradually to raise the level of functioning of the mind to the highest stage where it is ready for spiritual experience.

1. In order to raise the Mudha to the Ksipta level, simple physical exercises and elementary pranayama (breath control) are used. Physical activity, with some mental involvement, reduces mental agitation.

2. In the Ksipta stage the student is not confused, but s/he is still distracted and wavering. At this level pranayama and relaxation can help to achieve a certain steadiness of mind.

3. At the Viksipta level, where the mind is occasionally steady, relaxation, meditation, and visualisation are used to achieve some control over mental functioning.

4. At the Ekagra level there is the ability to control mental disturbances.

5. At the highest level of Niruddha there is peace of mind and spiritual enlightenment.

Mrs Bhava found that most of her patients were poor people who were attending the hospital in the hope of obtaining medicine and electric shock treatment. They belonged to either the Mudha or the Ksipta category. They were treated by yoga therapy on alternate days in groups of 5–10, the sessions lasting for ½–1 hour. They were expected to complete 12 sessions in the hospital and were told to do the practices at home on alternate days when they did not attend the hospital.

The sessions started with chanting and with yoga exercises comprising kriyas (cleansing techniques), asanas (postures), and pranayama – all of them simple and elementary. These were taught to all the patients irrespective of their mind level. Some of them did not want to sit quietly watching their breathing and preferred to sit watching the others, so certain modifications were made to suit individual needs. As the therapy progressed some patients were told to increase the duration of their pranayama when practising at home and also to practise pranayama if their symptoms should become worse at any time.

At the end of the 4-week period Mrs Bhava carried out post-therapy evaluation based partly on personal interviews with each patient, and partly on her observations during the course. Out of the 30 patients receiving therapy, 9 did not show proper application and failed to complete the course. Of the remaining 21 who completed the course to the Mrs Bhava's satisfaction, 11 belonged to the Mudha category and 10 to the Ksipta category, and the assessment in the individual categories was as follows:

	Mudha	Ksipta	Total
Marked progress	4	4	8
Moderate progress	5	4	9
Mild progress	1	0	1
No progress	1	2	3
Totals	11	10	21

Group Two – This group of thirty patients were given behaviour therapy of deep muscle relaxation based on the Jacobson's method. In this long-established therapy, the patient consciously tries to relax various muscle groups while lying down. The effectiveness of this technique is based on principles of learning theory and conditioning. The patients (who had already had experience of this method) were given the therapy intensive course three times on alternate days over the 4-week period. They were encouraged to practise it at home.

When the 4-week courses were over, the patients from both groups were seen by the Research Officer, and post-therapeutic evaluation was carried out by clinical methods and psychological testing by means of the Hamilton Behaviour Scales. It was found that 70 per cent of the yoga group and 76.6 per cent of the behaviour therapy group showed clinically significant improvement. As the latter group were already used to the treatment a better result was to be expected compared with the yoga group who were new to the therapy and had a very limited period in which to learn it. The results showed that yoga as a therapy works very well with the Ksipta level of patients and moderately well with the Mudha level. However, the hospital concluded that further confirmation was needed by well-controlled, long-term, follow-up studies.

Summary

Mrs Bhava told me that from the results of this comparative study she had gained more confidence in what she was doing with psychiatric patients. She was therefore keen to continue the Yoga, and the Dean of K.E.M. Hospital gave permission.

Mrs Bhava worked on a voluntary basis for four months, until payment for her services was at last authorised through the necessary channels. Since then, as the hospital's official yoga therapist she had been part of the hospital system, teaching for two hours three days a week, and dealing with some of the patients' physical complaints as well as their mental problems, in groups of 7–10 persons. She found that during the first month she could usually hold the patients' interest for a 15-minute session, after which they tended to get upset and complained of not being able to grasp or express their inner feelings. Therefore she decided that for the first month 15-minute sessions were long enough; however, by the third week the patients generally became more relaxed and friendly towards her. The length of the sessions was gradually increased up to 45 minutes by the twelfth week. Patients who originally just watched, eventually, in their own time, began to participate.

All the yoga techniques were taught in slow steps, so as to register fully in the patients' minds, and only then were they able to practise at home. Those who did, became more self-reliant and eager to help themselves.

Some of the patients came from some distance away, and Mrs Bhava asked them initially to attend three times a week for one month, to learn some basic yoga techniques which they could then practise at home. After that they were asked to return every six months so that their performance could be checked.

The techniques Mrs Bhava used under the guidance of Dr Jayadeva and Shri Ghurye of the Yoga Institute, Santa Cruz, covered a wide range of pranayamas, kriyas, asanas, and relaxation exercises, which were designed to help circulation, digestion, cleanliness, eating habits, to improve sleeping patterns, and engender enthusiasm and confidence in daily life. She said that most of her patients were glad to continue their yoga practices, with very satisfactory results.

Address:

The Yoga Institute, SANTA CRUZ (East), Bombay – 400 055.

CHAPTER TWELVE

Visits to the Ramana Iyengar Memorial Yoga Institute – medical classes

M y encounter with Yogacharya B.K.S. (Bellur Krishnamachar Sundararaja) Iyengar was the most startling experience of my whole Indian tour. Having since read his fascinating book 'Body the Shrine, Yoga Thy Light', I think I can understand from his account of his early life why his reception of me was so unfriendly, in fact positively hostile.

Iyengar was born in 1918, during a worldwide influenza epidemic, to a poor family with thirteen children of whom ten survived. Throughout his childhood he remained a sickly child with – as he describes himself – 'thin arms and legs, a protruding stomach, and a top-heavy head'. At the age of thirteen he suffered from malaria.

When Iyengar was about sixteen, one of his elder sisters married Shri T. Krishnamacharya, a first-class scholar and a Professor of Yoga. Shortly after their marriage, Iyengar went to live with them in Mysore. He recounts in his book how Krishnamacharya, although a kind-hearted man, was hot-tempered. Gradually this affected Iyengar to the point where he became too nervous and frightened even to stand or sit in Krishnamacharya's presence. Krishnamacharya always refused to teach Iyengar any yoga, telling him that he was unsuitable, a weakling, and it all stemmed from his karma (the law of cause and effect which claims handicaps in one's life are due to misdeeds committed in a previous one.) Nevertheless, Iyengar tried to do some asanas on his own, only to find that his body was 'as stiff as a poker'.

The Maharaja of Mysore was a keen student of philosophy and under the guidance of Krishnamacharya he realised the value of yoga. He engaged Krishnamacharya to teach yoga in the Palace's 'yogashala' (a room allocated to yoga) for the benefit of the royal family. Yet Krishnamacharya still would not teach Iyengar the asanas. It was not until a considerable time later, when one of the orphan boys whom he had trained as a yoga expert left the

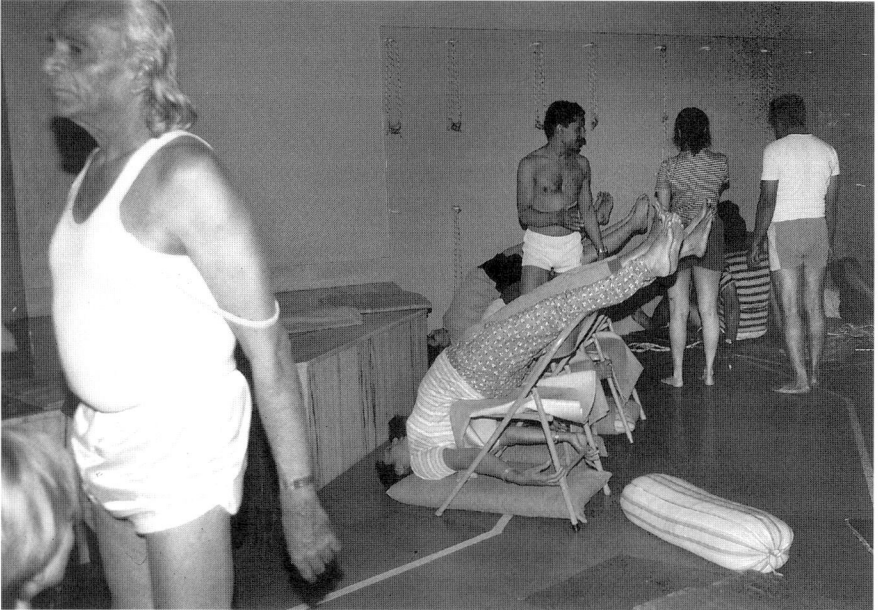

Yogacharya B.K.S. Iyengar.

Palace's demonstration team, that Krishnamacharya decided after all to teach Iyengar some asanas for one month only.

The year 1935 was the beginning of Iyengar's path in yoga, with Krishnamacharya initiating him into the traditional Thread Ceremony, accompanied by the Gayatri Mantra (Universal Sound of Prayer and Devotion). At the end of the course Iyengar and other boys gave a demonstration at the Palace. He was then chosen to teach asanas in the yogashala twice daily, early in the morning and after school in the evening. He states in his book that for years thereafter he taught and practised the asanas in a purely mechanical way, doggedly fulfilling his duties although his legs were very painful and his back ached almost unbearably. Because he was afraid of his teacher, he felt he could not reveal his difficulties and unhappiness to anyone.

In spite of his early years of struggle, he has since pursued his single-minded devotion to yoga, achieving a deep understanding of the asanas which has enabled him to teach yoga successfully to many eminent people, as well as to others all over the world. In December 1974, the Ramana Iyengar Memorial Yoga Institute was established, named in honour of his beloved wife Ramani who had recently died. Ever since, his daughter Geeta and his son Prashant have also devoted their lives to yoga. Geeta took to practising yoga when she was a young child because she suffered from nephritis, and yoga cured her.

Ten years later, in December 1984, Chris and I arrived for our prearranged visit to the Iyengar medical classes, which took place for one session on Tuesdays and Wednesdays each week. The evening before our visit, I rang the Institute to inform Geeta of our arrival. She told me the time of the medical class session the next day.

We duly arrived at the Institute, a magnificent three-tier building described in Iyengar's book as constructed in the shape of a circular pyramid supported by eight columns. The medical class took place in the main hall where many large photographs were displayed of Iyengar performing complicated asanas. Just before the class was due to begin, Iyengar stormed in refusing to address me, but shouting to Chris, 'She cannot attend this class, because she has not done my course and will not understand what I am doing'. I took courage from the letter Geeta had written in reply to me four months previously welcoming me to attend the medical classes. Iyengar glared at me exclaiming, 'You think you can come here and learn in one lesson'. I protested, 'But Mr Iyengar, I attended Iyengar yoga classes in London for three years back in the early seventies'. At this point Geeta took command and came over to greet me. Iyengar lowered his voice, complaining to her, but then accepted the situation since his daughter had invited me earlier and took the responsibility. He said grudgingly that it would be all right for us to stay to watch the medical classes, but we were on no account to ask questions or interrupt the class in any way. He instructed Geeta to take me around the class and explain the various problems of the pupils.

There were about twenty pupils, most of them Indian. Geeta gave me a quick rundown of their complaints, as follows: headaches and migraine, asthma, jaundice, circulatory problems, menstruation problems, anxiety and neurosis, hypertension and high blood pressure, angina, rheumatism and arthritis, spondylitis, diabetes, obesity, facial paralysis, paralysis in both legs, polio, scoliosis and other spinal deformities and injuries – quite a formidable list!

There were almost as many helpers as pupils. The helpers were trained in India, Australia and the West in Iyengar's yoga methods, and were now learning his medical techniques. As soon as the class began, Iyengar focused his full attention on his pupils' particular needs and instructed his helpers how to help support and manipulate the pupils into various poses.

Equipment consisted of blue yoga mats, blankets and pieces of carpet, bolsters, disc-shaped pads, stools, folding chairs, bars, a variety of wooden blocks, buckled straps, ropes, looped rope with weights, ropes and hooks in the wall, a vaulting-horse, wooden frames with holes down the sides wide enough for ropes to be fed through, metal bars with sections of rubber padding attached and finally small silk-covered bean bags. No wonder Iyengar referred to this hall as his 'torture chamber'!

It was fascinating to watch the action as Iyengar yelled at the pupils who were being pushed, pulled, propped up and held securely in position with the aid of various pieces of equipment (which appeared to me to be an extension of the manual equipment used in physiotherapy). Iyengar, Geeta and Prashant moved swiftly around the hall teaching each pupil highly sophisticated physiother-apeutic yoga techniques. I witnessed pupils being forcibly levered and manipulated into postures by methods I had never dreamed of, and Iyengar's approach was certainly the most dynamic and strenuous form of body control that I had ever seen. I could well understand why he was one of the most famous teachers of yoga in the world today, and why his system was a specialist occupation.

Towards the end of the session, the yelling from Iyengar and the bustle of activity quietened down, and the pupils relaxed. Then gradually they departed, not limp and exhausted as one might have expected, but glowing with satisfaction. Iyengar himself disappeared down a spiral staircase. I thanked Geeta warmly and confirmed our return for the medical class the following day.

I left the Institute eager to know more about these complex contortion postures, and to experience for myself what such pos-tures felt like. Back in our hotel, Chris and I discussed the overwhelming activity we had witnessed and talked about Iyengar's rudeness to me. Chris believed that although Iyengar's initial verbal attack on me had been most unpleasant, there was a much greater depth to this man than had emerged at our meeting and that this depth would eventually surface above the superficial turbulence. For my part, I really did not want to leave Pune with memories only of this aggressive yoga master and without any real grasp of his medical yoga techniques. We therefore agreed that I should write to him and ask if we might attend an intensive yoga course with him at the Institute. I posted the letter through his letter-box early next morning.

Later that day, when we arrived to attend our second medical class, we found Iyengar hanging upside down supported by suspended ropes interlaced round the thighs and ankles. He came down, extricated himself from the entanglement and immediately began the lesson.

He gave me a curt nod indicating that I could take photographs and I took full advantage of the permission. The only words Iyengar said to us that day were, 'You see, it is not the yoga that makes these people do the postures, it is my personality'. At the end of the session he again disappeared down his spiral staircase. It was his Registrar who informed us of his decision that I myself could attend a three-week intensive yoga course with Iyengar, but that Chris would not be able to join any course at the Institute, as they were all fully booked. However, I decided that to leave Chris out, when he had put himself at my disposal to travel with me and do all the videoing, was out of the question. I therefore wrote again to Iyengar, asking if he would allow us to return in three weeks' time to video the whole of a medical class for showing back in the UK. Fortunately he gave his permission.

During our final visit to Iyengar's medical class, a reporter and photographer from the local newspaper were present and they were allowed to ask Iyengar any questions while he was conducting the class. He took them round with him from one pupil to another, explaining why each was doing that particular technique. This was

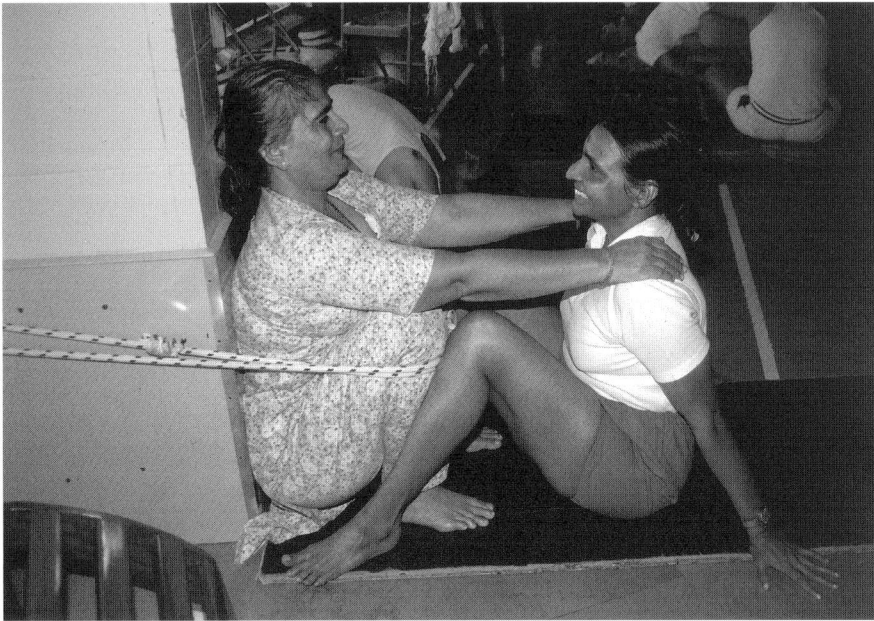

Geeta Iyengar (right) assisting pupil.

in marked contrast to his attitude to Chris and myself – although I must add that throughout Geeta gave us her best attention.

In any event, Chris was able to video sixty minutes of the class activities, which clearly showed the efficacy of his medical class methods. To give some insight into his approach, here is a maxim from the 'Learning and Teaching' section in his book, p. 249: 'Give a hint, and nothing happens, give a hit, and see what happens!' During the session Iyengar remarked, 'These westerners, they complain of pain so much, but we Indians are not afraid of pain. The westerners think if their knee hurts, it's a fracture, and if they hear a click, that's a fracture – they don't know the difference between a click and a fracture!'

At the end of the session I asked Iyengar if he would grant me an interview, and he replied, 'I am too tired and hungry, I've been up working since very early this morning, and it is now 8 p.m.' He then disappeared, leaving me with so many questions. His Registrar advised me to return at 10 a.m. next morning. I could speak with him then.

We arrived at 9.45 a.m. and found Iyengar striding through the grounds. I took my courage in both hands and asked if he would grant me one last favour and allow me to interview him. At that point a car arrived to pick him up, and he said as he got in, 'I have an important appointment to keep, come back at five and

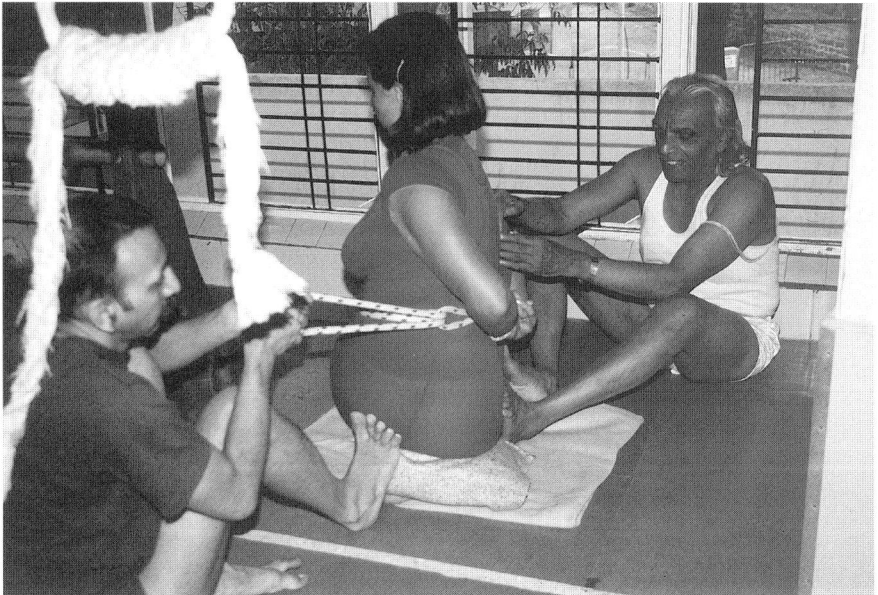

Mr Iyengar and helper assisting a Western patient into posture.

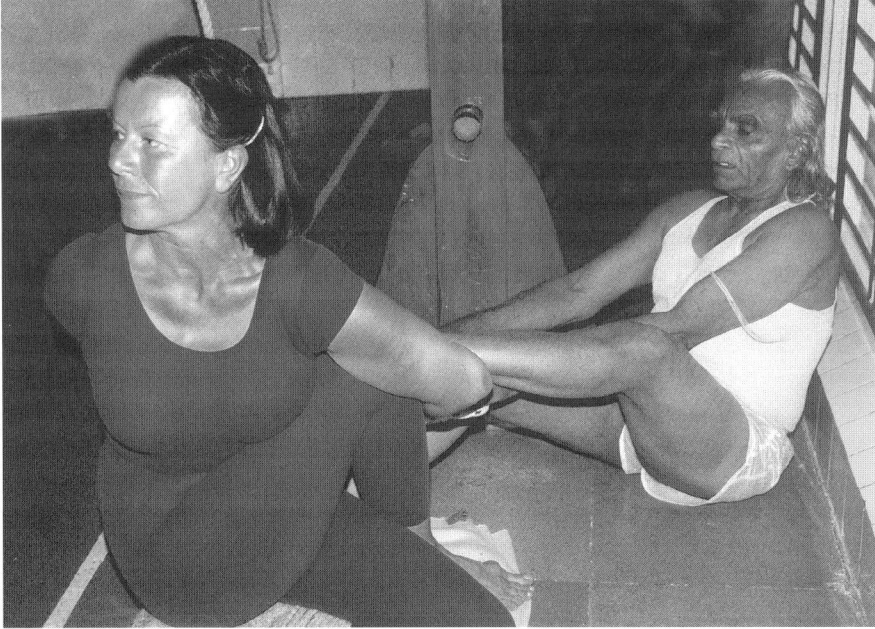

Achieving Ardha Matsyendra (Full Abdominal Twist).

I'll do it then.' I pleaded, 'But Mr Iyengar, I have a flight booked for 6.30 tonight' – but he snapped, '5 o'clock or not at all,' and off he went. I was determined to keep the appointment and collect what information I could in the short time available.

I was anxious to find out why his yoga system was so successful and seemed to be taking precedence over all others, including the traditional yoga system. This success was in spite of the fact that his own system was highly specialised, concentrating on body exercises mainly, with little reference to other forms of yoga.

At 5 p.m. we duly arrived in an auto-rickshaw, complete with all our luggage and video equipment. Iyengar greeted us in a much more friendly fashion and reciprocated my use of the traditional Namaste greeting (placing the palms together and bowing the head). He led us into his library where we were confronted by a skeleton in a display cabinet. I asked if he used this skeleton in his teaching but he answered, 'No. What is there is dead matter, and not like the real body that we work with. I teach with my live body, and use the pupils' faculties to show how asana can be done, whereas the medical profession study dead flesh and bones, then give patients examinations with instruments, and finally prescribe a drug to help cure the body.'

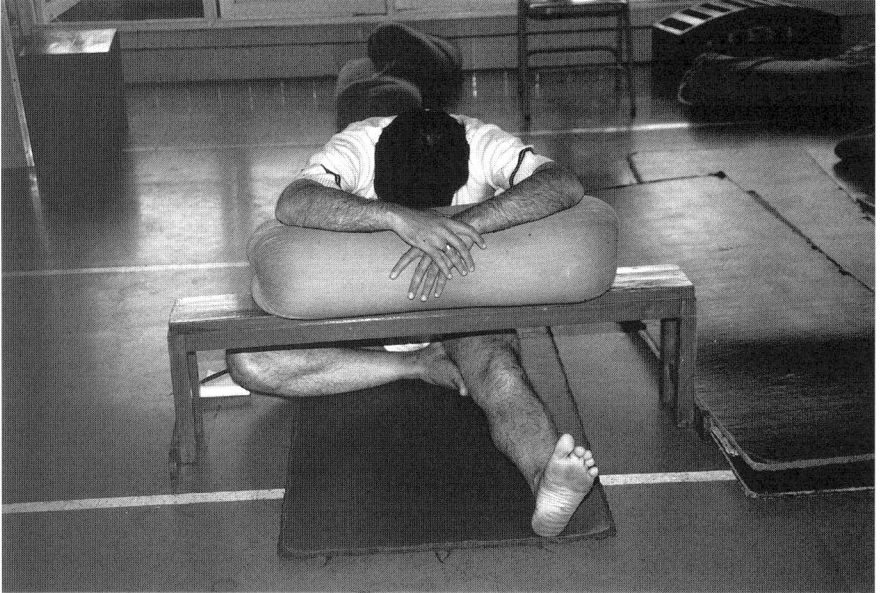
Quietening down in Janusirasana.

'How do you see consciousness developing in yoga?' I asked.

'Where is mind?' he replied. 'It is everywhere we think it is, and consciousness develops through the mind. Through yoga we can know what is inside ourselves. The body is part of the consciousness, and in yoga we become aware of our body and our breath. It is like the ocean, with the waves along the shoreline coming in contact with the sand on the beach. This is similar to the air we breathe which comes in contact with the cells in the body. The same force is behind the waves which flow in a forever changing pattern along the shoreline, as the life force in the mind, and the two are equally unpredictable. It is from that life force that consciousness is developed. There is no piece of scientific equipment that matches equipment of the human mind. The conscious mind can move anywhere, any time, anyhow, any way. As leaves move in the wind, your mind moves with your breath. If you understand how to distribute Prana, you can bring about the union of the energies of the individual and of the universe.

'No one can measure the extent of a person's physical pain, emotional disturbance, spiritual difficulties, or happiness, except through the practice of yoga. One comes in contact with the intelligence of the cells by movement of the mind throughout the body. To prove the worth of yoga is the job of the yogi who practises it; only when he can do this does yoga become a Science for the Self. The practitioner of yoga can maintain an even balance through all the disturbances and suffering of daily life.

He went on, 'Today everything is outside ourselves, therefore a great deal of awareness is discovered through the body. I think the old traditional practices of yoga should be left behind in the olden times when man's environment and situation allowed him to be introspective and resistant to the outer. That is why I work on the body.'

Needless to say, I did not agree with this view, having proved over and over again the efficacy of the traditional system of yoga in developing the person on a threefold basis of body, mind and spirit. However, I was certainly not going to argue with him for I wished to elicit his views to the greatest extent possible.

I asked him, 'Do you think there is a difference between PE exercises and yoga postures?'

He replied, 'Yes, because in PE only one part of the body is exercised. For instance in tennis only the parts of the body needed to play tennis are used, while other parts of the body remain unused. If the person is right-handed he is strong on the right but cannot function properly the left. But in yoga we use both hands and both sides of the body; we use what could be called holistic exercises, because there is nothing neglected, from the skin to the self and from the self to the skin. That is the difference.'

'Would you care to comment on your medical yoga classes?' I asked.

'As far as I know, there are two ways of treating disease. One is natural and the other is artificial, yet both work together with nature. When the doctor gives medicine to the patient, it is in order to invigorate nature to work with greater speed, and it does succeed in making dormant nature work a little better. This means that nature itself is the real healer, and yoga is entirely a natural method, where we use our own inner resources to fight the attacking disease.

'In our teachings we pay tremendous attention to the circulation, because circulation is the only thing which feeds the entire cells. Electricity is produced only when there is a tremendous flow of water in a tremendous velocity from the top to the bottom, and in the same way the bio-energy in the body has to be produced to increase our circulation in various ways. That is why there are so many asanas that bring the blood to the affected areas thus generating the power to heal.'

My next question was, 'What qualifications does a person need to work like yourself in a medical class?'

Iyengar said, 'The qualification is that he or she should be a perfect practitioner with a perfect understanding of the anatomy of the postures – not the anatomy of the actual body, because the asana *is* the anatomy, and we must know precisely which asana works on which part of the body. I think such people are then capable of helping the suffering.

'Yoga is a healing science, and here we bring out the weak points of each individual in order to break the habitual diseases which come to him through non-attention. We develop certain habits, and these habits cause what are called 'habitual diseases'. These habitual diseases are dependent on the five elements of the body, i.e. earth, air, fire, water, and ether, of which our bodies consist. If the radiation of any one of these is stronger than the others, there is sickness. It is the same with nature: if there is no disturbance of the natural seasons, everything in the environment is plentiful, but if the rain does not arrive at the right time, then there is an imbalance, so that the farmer needs water in order to plough. Similarly in the human body, imbalances are very frequent, e.g. constipation is because the element of earth is stronger than the other elements. With people suffering from swelling due to fluid accumulation, their water element is stronger. If people get a burning sensation in the stomach, eyes, chest, etc., their fire element is stronger. If they suffer from flatulence, bloated sensations, and rheumatoid arthritis involving painful swelling their ether element is stronger.'

I asked Mr Iyengar how this worked.

He replied, 'Ether creates space. Of course, there is no actual fluid here, there is just swelling. Space can be created both inside and outside – that is the quality of ether. So, to sum up, an imbalance due to our habits will increase and bring on disease. Yoga works to correct the five elements through balancing them in the body in the right proportions, so that one is immune to disease. Thus yoga is a curative and healing process.'

I asked him if he thought yoga was necessary for complete healing.

He replied, 'Naturally, if you do not sleep you do not have

enough energy, because the brain needs rest. But we have got some poses in yoga which give the brain a certain supply of blood so that you feel as though you have slept. Therefore the process of rejuvenation is faster through the practice of yoga. No other system in the world has this influence on rejuvenation, which is why I can say that yoga is superior to all other forms of exercise.'

I asked, 'Mr Iyengar, do you see the poor people throughout the world benefiting from yoga?'

He replied to my surprise, 'My dear friend, I know that nutrition is tremendously important in a poor country like India, where the majority of people cannot get enough to eat and their aim is just to survive. In such a situation you cannot keep on at people about the value of nourishment. In India there is no choice, they have to make do with whatever is available. In your affluent country everything is available, so you are all right; even though there is stress and strain, you can choose food according to your taste and needs. In my country, and in Africa, where the standard of living is low, what yoga can do for the inhabitants is to increase the circulatory system so as to help them to digest whatever food they eat. This helps them to resist disease. Therefore yoga is of assistance to both the undernourished and the overnourished. Malnutrition can be made good by what I call biofeedback – an adjustment in the strengths of the various parts of the body to help maintain it in reasonable health. In short, yoga is a gateway for improving the respiratory and circulatory systems. Yoga speaks also of the pranayama and of the postures. The former is vital energy, and the latter deals with functions of the body that are stimulated by the circulatory exercises. If both these aspects are working together in harmony, good health results.'

Time was up. I thanked Iyengar for a very helpful and illuminating discourse. He smiled and thanked me in return. We parted on far better terms than those which had marred our first encounter.

I felt I had gained some understanding of the theories, as well as the practice, of a remarkable man of worldwide reputation, but naturally I could not help regretting his – to my mind – overemphasis of the bodily aspects of a system which to me is a complete guide to the fullness of life in all its aspects.

Conclusion

I learnt from Iyengar that a full understanding of the postures is essential in yoga therapy and that the yoga postures can be modified to the individual's abilities. Iyengar reinforced in me that it is not the yoga that makes people do the postures, as he said 'It is my personality'.

In other words, when students have confidence in and respect for their yoga trainer, they will give their best cooperation to learn what is being taught to them. This is what is necessary in teaching yoga before progress can be made. However, it does take time for trainers to develop their skills and knowledge in a yoga system and only through practice and study is it possible for trainers to develop the necessary personal qualities for establishing good relationships with their students. Then the scope is limitless, providing there is understanding of the mechanics of the techniques used, together with the right intention to benefit the student.

Reference: B.K.S. Iyengar, *Body the Shrine, Yoga Thy Light*, published by B.I. Taraporewala (Bombay, 1978).

Address:
Ramana Iyengar Memorial Yoga Institute, 1107 – B/1, Shivaji Nagar, PUNE – 411 016.

CHAPTER THIRTEEN

Dr Bandorawalla's Leprosy Hospital

A former Churchill Fellow, Gina Levete, founder of 'Interlink' (Integration through the Arts), advised me to see Mohan Agashe who lived in Pune. When we arrived there, I contacted him, and learned that he was a well known actor as well as a qualified psychiatrist. He told me he had started using drama-creativity, combined with yoga exercises, with some psychiatric patients at the Sasoon Hospital in Pune, to very good effect. His life was one of thriving activity, and he was certainly an entertaining personality.

When Mohan Agashe learned about my fellowship he suggested I should meet his friend Dr Rajiv Sharangpani, a well known cricketer. Dr Sharangpani was a consultant in Sports Medicine, and also a surgeon operating on disabled people at the Leprosy Hospital.

For a change from the usual sober venue, we all gathered in an American-style ice-cream bar. Dr Sharangpani turned out to be a very interesting person. As well as being a general surgeon, he had studied Sports Medicine in West Germany. For more than fifteen years he had regularly practised yoga and he claimed that this was the reason why he had never suffered injuries from playing cricket, whereas the other players came to him with ankle and knee problems. He showed them some yoga movements to loosen-up those joints and the results had been extremely encouraging. He discovered that the combination of yoga postures, which can make the body supple, with sport medicine to make the muscles work in their full range, helped to tone up the soft tissue and ligaments – the main complaint of the cricketers. Dr Sharangpani was writing a book for children, from babyhood to teenage, to incorporate these ideas.

Dr Sharangpani invited us to his house to meet his wife and two children. He showed us a set of slides of himself demonstrating what looked like advanced yoga postures, while he described the similarity of the yoga techniques to those of Sports Medicine.

Next day he took us 13 kms to visit the Dr Bandorawalla Leprosy

Hospital where he was conducting experiments for the 'body-image' of men, women and children who were suffering from leprosy. The hospital was a very large well organised building of modern architecture and technology, surrounded by immaculately built native huts for the rehabilitation patients' living quarters. The patients had built these huts themselves in the hospital grounds, and there was a real community spirit among them. The hospital's 400 beds were always filled with patients from all over India. Dr Sharangpani said, 'Some patients arrive with advanced leprosy, while some are in the early stages merely suffering from ulcers which are not such severe problems. But, however crowded we are, since they have travelled so far we have to admit them and give them treatment before sending them back.' The hospital is supported by Poona (Pune) District Leprosy Committee, Infirmary Block, 1977; International Foundation (through Lions Club of Poona Kirta), USA; and Help the Aged, UK.

Leprosy is a severe disease which affects the bones, skin, mucous membranes and nerves. The causative organism is Mycobacterium Leprae. Nowadays it is only slightly contagious; most people being naturally immune. If it is treated early enough with chemotherapy and physiotherapy, it can be corrected and normal function restored, but if it is not treated in time, the destruction of the nerves leads to deformities. These include foot-drop, wrist-drop, claw-foot, extensive ulceration of extremities leading to loss of fingers and toes, and absorbtion of bone affecting the nose, eyes, and larynx. However, plastic orthopaedic surgery can treat chronic leprosy invalidism and enable the patient to return to the community and lead a reasonably active life.

Dr Sharangpani said, 'Before and after surgery we use Sports Medicine, in which the patients work with various aids and apparatus to develop muscle strength. Basically the muscle exercise is to develop the agonist as well as the antagonist muscles, that is, extend both the front and back muscles with an equal amount of exercise. Also we try to disabuse patients of the idea that their bodies are something 'dirty' which has gone wrong, and we encourage them to have a positive approach to life.

'The area on which we are going to operate must first undergo a process of straightening the joints and strengthening the muscles. Then after surgery we continue the process of strengthening the surrounding muscles which will have to take over the functions of the parts that have been removed. The developing of these muscles will increase the patient's strength, endurance and flexibility.'

When leprosy affected the hands, fingers and thumbs, it made the fingers and thumbs stiffen and bend inwards. Before surgery the affected fingers were straightened by the application of plaster-of-paris splints round each finger, which were changed every other day, gradually straightening out the joints until they become completely straight. Only then could surgery be carried out to remove the affected part.

The series of exercises to strengthen the fingers were:

1. The screwing up of a sheet of newspaper in the hand – one hand at a time. This enabled all the fingers to work the full range of joint movements necessary in ordinary working life. Dr Sharangpani told us, 'The screwing up of a sheet of paper in one hand was used by people who practice the old martial art of Krishna Vidya. When patients use their right hand to screw up the paper, similar movements simultaneously occur involuntarily in the opposite hand. This is called 'the crossing effect'. This exercise is used for one hand when the other is in plaster, so that similar motor action can be achieved more easily by the inactive hand when the plaster is removed.'

2. The moulding of plasticine into a ball by the thumb and fingers of one hand. This exercise was used when the thumb was not rotating in its full 90-degree range which would affect the functioning of the whole hand. Later, the patient had to mould the plasticine to form human figures. Comparison of these figures over a period showed the improvement in finger dexterity.

3. Moving two or three small chrome balls around in the hand as quickly as possible. This trained the fingers to move with the speed which is necessary in daily life.

Dr Sharangpani said that when leprosy affected the mobility of the feet and toes, the ankle was unable to lift the foot from the ground. To correct this the patient was given an external spring attached from his knee to his shoe. This helped the knee to lift the ankle so that the foot could clear the ground and the patient could walk after a fashion; but surgery was subsequently carried out to enable him to walk normally without any aids. Usually this was done by replacing the interior muscle above the ankle by another tendon, although in advanced cases it might be necessary to amputate the limb.

In all cases, both before and after surgery, patients had to strengthen the front and back surrounding muscles. Some of the exercises performed were:

4. To develop the front muscles of the thigh the patient sat on a piece of apparatus like a vaulting-horse which had a bar at chest level as well as at foot level. He placed his feet under the bar at foot level and levered it up and down several times.

    To develop the hamstring muscles in the back of the thighs he lay face downwards on top of the horse with his hands clasped behind his back, placed his feet under the top bar and levered it up and down several times.

5. To develop the thigh muscles when the patient's legs and feet were in plaster, he lay on his back on a flat surface and perform leg-lifting movements, so that when the plaster was removed the muscle strength had been maintained. Otherwise the weakened state of the muscles would mean an increase in the rehabilitation period.

    Some patients were able gradually to increase their endurance until they could lift the heavy weight of the leg-plaster up to 100 times.

6. To strengthen the back and abdominal muscles the patient first lay downwards on a couch with his hands clasped behind his neck. A physiotherapist held his thighs to support him firmly, while he performed lifting up his trunk several times. He then turned over on his back and performed lift ups from that position.

In cases where the leprosy had caused the nasal bridge to sink owing to destruction of the nasal cartilage, the cartilage was completely removed and the patients were given a new nose fitting. One patient showed us how he could take his nose fitting out to clean it and then put it back himself, and he had become so used to it that it seemed like a part of his body. Dr Sharangpani said, 'The surgery has made his nose absolutely all right, and the difference in his personality is remarkable. All patients do extremely well here, and we intend to publish medical papers on our activities.'

There were children at the hospital, some of whom had leprosy and others were the children of mothers who were being treated. A one-hour yoga class was held twice a week for women and children, conducted by a teacher from Iyengar's Institute who had been coming regularly for two years. She said, 'When we started, the students were incapacitated, and could not stay long in one posture, but they have now come on so far that they can hold most of the poses for quite some time. Sometimes because of their disability they may say that they are very tired, or their head aches, or their legs ache, and I then make them do the standing postures against the wall. If they have stomach ache, I make them lie on benches. I have found a definite improvement in their health over the past two years, so naturally I enjoy teaching them.'

Dr Sharangpani told us that there were two types of training at the hospital; one was physical training to strengthen the flexibility of the patients' limbs and the other was to restore their working capacity. The latter was done by giving them some vocational training, so that when they had to leave the hospital they could earn their living through a trade. Illiteracy was also a problem because most of the patients were from the lower economic strata, and educational facilities were provided to teach them to read and write. Vocational training included dairy and poultry farming, and there was also an engineering unit. All the hospital workers were in fact leprosy patients.

The physiotherapist, a young man called Anjendi, continued our

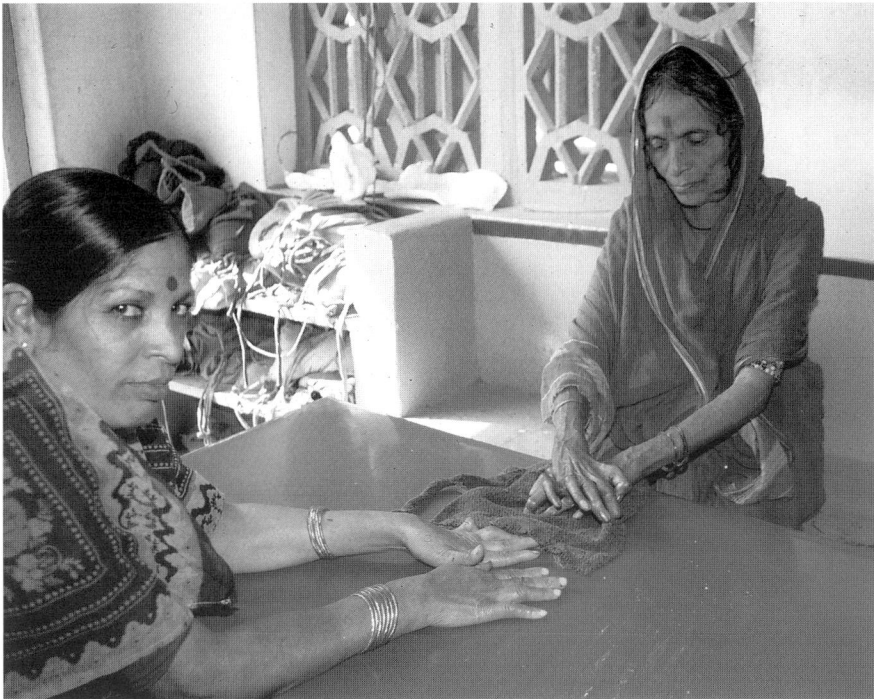

Patients massage their hands with oil.

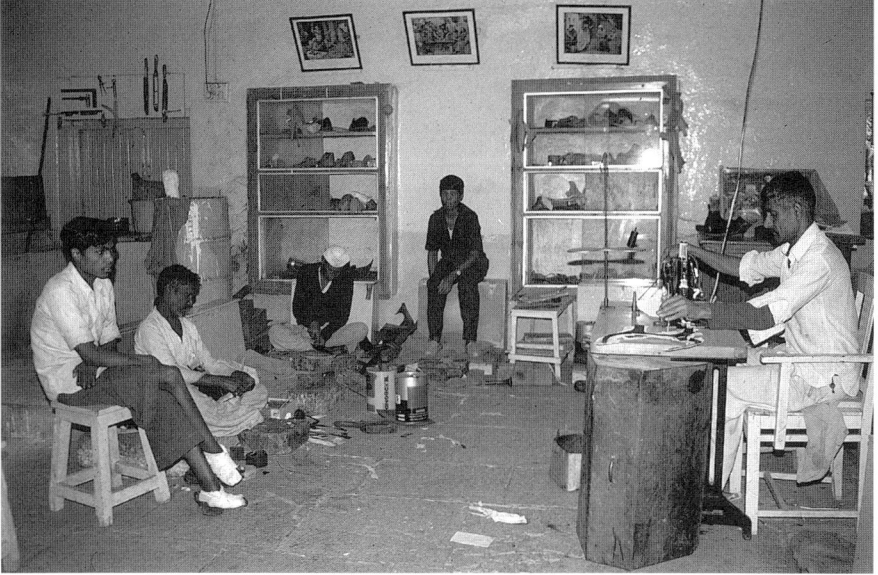

Unit where physio-aids are made for patients' footwear.

tour of the hospital by showing us some other vocational facilities. He took us round the unit where physio-aids were being made for the patients' footwear; the unit where they massaged their hands with oil; the loom section where they were making bandages and dusters; the hospital's communal kitchen where everybody's food was prepared; and the training section in tailoring. Anjendi told us that the hospital arranged a bank loan for those who had completed their apprentice training so that they could buy a sewing machine to start their own business when they left hospital. This project had proved very successful and one ex-patient had extended his business to employ six other people and supply each of them with a sewing machine.

Anjendi told us that all the buildings in the grounds, which were made of cemented brick and stone with roofs of thatch or corrugated iron, were built by the patients. A recent addition to the hospital was a solar heating system which supplied the patients' quarters and communal kitchens with constant hot water and electricity. Another addition was a bio-gas tank utilising cow dung and human excrement to produce heating power for cooking in the kitchens and sterilising surgical instruments.

Anjendi impressed us greatly by explaining about himself in excellent English. His right hand had no fingers owing to his previous leprosy, and he told us that before he contracted the

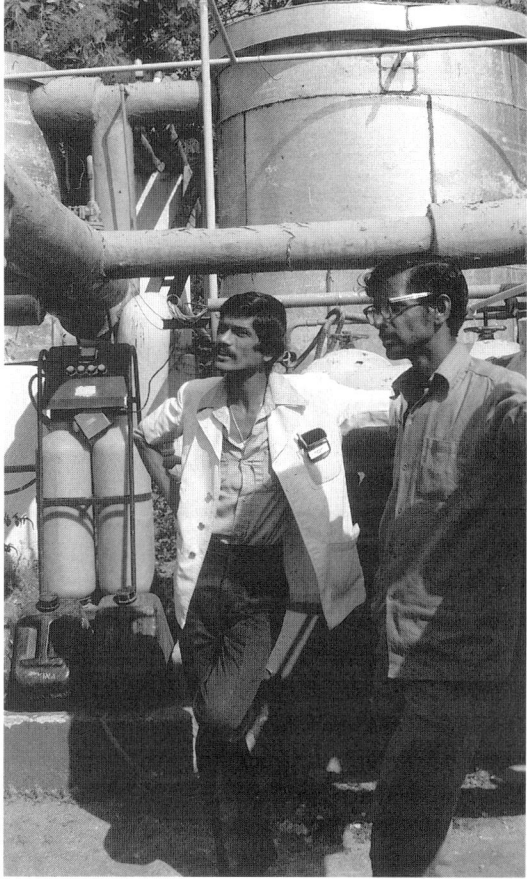

Anjendi (left) standing in front of
the bio-gas tank.

disease he was studying engineering and was a television artist in
his spare time. He had to give this up when he contracted the
disease, and he said, 'At that time I felt that because I could not
do anything I could not live, but by the grace of Almighty I came
to this hospital and now I am cured. When that happened this
institute sent me to Madras District Medical College where I trained
in physiotherapy. I am now a member of the medical staff here,
earning a wage and very happy in my independence. I am able to
give help to others by showing them that I can do things even
without my hand, and I aim to teach them that they can do the
same.' Another living example of victory over adversity, who rejoiced
in telling us that he had recently married a healthy young woman
and was now even happier because they had a healthy baby boy.

Address:
Bandorawalla Leprosy Hospital, Kondhawa Budruk, PUNE – 411 022.

CHAPTER FOURTEEN

At Ram Krishna Vivekananda Yog Ashram, Aligarh, with Ram Autar Sharma

After meeting Mr Sharma at the YOCOCEN Conference, we visited his centre in Aligarh, and saw the therapeutic work carried out for the local community by him and Miss Bharti. They had worked together since 1971 and had been successful in curing the following ailments: constipation, high blood pressure, asthma, sinusitis, arthritis, cervical spondylitis, backache, a diabetes, nervous tension, headache and migraine, obesity, menstrual disorders, and others.

Mr Sharma and Miss Bharti taught separately at the Aligarh Muslim University, and they arranged meetings and yoga demonstrations for us in the various departments of the men's and women's sections. We were very interested to note how keen some of the students were to attend yoga classes twice a week in their own time.

Miss A. Thomas, the Principal of the University, told us that not all the students were Muslims. She was a Catholic and the university was a multi-religious and cultural society. She said that the women's section were trying to bring their level of education and opportunity up to that of the men, in accordance with the system operating in the west.

Mrs Amino Kishore, a teacher of English, took us to meet some students and tutors in the Art and Psychology Departments and the Career Planning Centre. We had a most enjoyable tour watching the deployment of the same skills and techniques as are used in the west.

We next attended a meeting at Mr Sharma's Centre where, at his request I gave a talk, with slides, on my yoga classes for people with learning disabilities in England. The Provost of the Psychology Department, then decided that in future yoga should be an extramural course in the University's curriculum for students wishing to work with the disabled – a very satisfactory outcome of my demonstration.

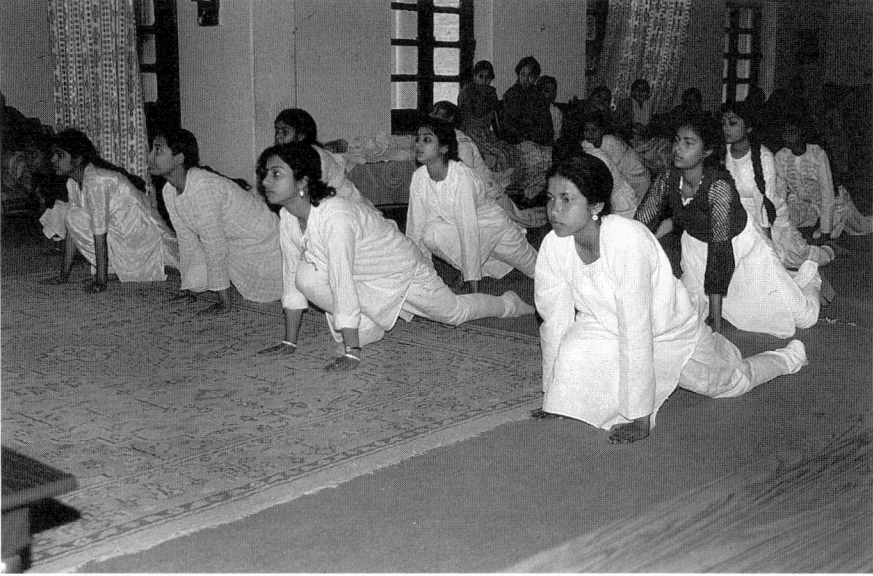

The women's yoga class.

Later we met Mr Naseem Waris, the General Secretary of Uttar Pradesh Disabled Association, Dharampur Castle, Maris Road, Aligarh, which was registered in 1981. Sadly, in 1974 he lost both legs in a train accident. He had previously been an expert horse-rider – a champion in 1968 – and after the accident his main aim was to resume riding. He was sent a pair of artificial legs from England and with perseverance and dedication, he learned how to use them to grip the sides of a horse – an achievement which gave him immense satisfaction. He told us that he had been fortunate enough to receive a special blessing from Mother Teresa for his courage and the good work he was able to do for disabled people. At this time, the association was working on a plan to set up a rehabilitation unit. The idea was to organise a town for disabled people, which they would run themselves, with special training to develop their aptitudes.

Mr Naseem Waris was very interested in my work and wanted me to stay longer to talk to his members. Unfortunately I had to refuse as the time for our departure was drawing near. I was pleased that he also decided to start regular yoga sessions for the members. He said he hoped that people like myself from the West would keep in touch with his association, to foster good relations and the exchange of suggestions, ideas and research for the benefit of disabled people.

The next appointment Mr Sharma had arranged for us was with his brother-in-law, Dr Kashmir Singh, Superintendent of Police at Aligarh. We met him at home with his family, who provided refreshments and a warm welcome. He told us that he had had a stiff neck problem due to his type of work, and he had asked Mr Sharma to teach him some yoga to deal with it. The exercises prescribed gave him instant relief and he had continued to practise them every day. He was now feeling much better and quite free from tension and neck pain. Here was one more sufferer who proved for himself the efficacy of yoga as a cure for health problems.

Mr Sharma then took us to the Gandhi Eye Hospital to meet the eye physician and surgeon, Dr J.M. Pahwa. We were steered to him through a large room thronged by about a hundred patients who parted before us to give us passage. Dr Pahwa greeted us with warm interest and enthusiasm and after a short talk with us said he would now look into ways in which yoga could help his patients suffering from eyestrain!

We were taken up two floors to Mr Sharma's workroom where he manufactured models of the head, the brain and the eye for medical students to study, and practised his profession of 'Eye Artistry'. He had been working in this field at the eye hospital since 1957 and was apparently the only person in India who still practised the profession. He had learnt this skill from the original founder of the hospital over a period of three years. He said, 'Eye Artistry involves looking into the eye through an opthalmoscope to see the retina, and painting a picture of the exact colours and shapes I find. At first I was amazed to see so many colours inside the eye. The art lies in mixing the water colours to get them exactly right before I start painting and it takes three days to complete a picture.'

Some of the finished paintings were on display, and showed the following eye disorders: retinal disease, papilloedema, retinal cyst cysticercus cellulose, macular dedema, Eales' disease, thrombosis of superior nasal branch of central vein.

Mr Sharma described how his Eye Artistry diagnoses were useful with his yoga students. He said, 'What we see is connected to the brain via the optic nerve, and it is that which is interpreted by the mind. The eye reveals some physical and mental weaknesses. For instance, if I see in a yoga student's eyes that his arteries are thin and could haemorrhage, I advise him not to do Sirshasana (head stand). I give the same advice to students who have high myopic vision (extreme near-sightedness) heart trouble, high blood pressure, diabetes, or hypertension.'

It was fascinating to see the paintings illustrating just what to look out for, with a view to use by both yoga teachers and medical students for preventative and educational purposes. Mr Sharma finished by showing us another masterpiece, a cross section of a life-size model of the head which had the bones, muscles, sinews, veins and arteries etc., painted on it in true colours. We thought it a splendid piece of artistry and educational work.

Mr Sharma gave me a copy of a recent paper he had written on osteo-arthritis which stated that yoga played an indirect role in managing this crippling disease. He had found that many patients who did not respond to conventional therapy improved through practising various yoga asanas. He concluded that the exact role of yoga in this condition would require long-term observation and follow-up of cases.

The results he had obtained over ten years were as follows:

	Numbers	Success	Failure	Drop-out
Arthritis of the extremities	89	80	4	5
Cervical spondylitis	96	85	5	6
Backache	132	120	10	2
Diabetes	185	125	25	35

Mr Sharma said, 'Many cases of diabetes – so often a cause of blindness – had been cured by yoga and this was recorded in a number of medical and scientific publications.' His conclusion was that certain yoga postures regularly practised pressed and stimulated the ailing pancreas gland from within. Diet was also an important part of the treatment. The yogic breathing exercises enlarged the breathing capacity of the middle and upper part of the lungs, with beneficial effect.

Finally, at the end of our two very interesting days in Aligarh, Mr Sharma performed, for us to video, the following typical session of pranayama as taught in his centre.

Note: It is advisable to be taught the following under the guidance of an expert.

1. Standing, breathe in through nose and raise arms, then breathe out through nose and lower arms. Repeat several times, as often as is comfortable. This stimulates the brain and sinus.

2.   a. Standing, raise arms in front of chest, start to breathe through mouth

b. Swing both arms to one side while breathing out through nose

c. Bring arms to front and inhale through mouth

d. Swing arms round to other side, exhaling through nose.

This is a technique which stimulates the respiration, circulation, brain and sinus.

3. Jumping, lift arms up while inhaling through mouth, and as feet come down exhale through nose, and lowering arms. Repeat about five times. This can relieve sinus trouble and colds, and can help to improve memory.

4. *Bhastrika Pranayama* – energetic techniques of breathing rapidly, with emphasis on exhalation.

These techniques should be used with caution.

i. Standing or sitting, lean head back and breathe in and out dynamically through the nose.
This technique oxygenates the head.

ii. Sit in Padmasana (Lotus posture, or sit comfortably). Use forefinger to close alternate nostrils, breathe in through the mouth, and out forcefully through each nostril. This cleanses the nasal passage in preparation for the next Bhastrika technique.

iii. Sitting, close right nostril with right thumb, and practice rapid (Bhastrika) breathing in and out with left nostril. Repeat conversely. Do the double exercise about twelve times. This can vitalise each side of the body in turn.

iv. Advanced Bhastrika (alternate nostril breathing). Close each nostril in turn with thumb or forefinger and breathe in rapidly through one nostril and out forcefully through the other. Then breathe in through the latter nostril and out through the other. Repeat as often as is comfortable. The complete practice of Bhastrika can energise the entire inside of the body.

Mr Sharma said, 'In the realm of yoga we relate the left nostril to the cool moon, and this left side is called the 'ida nadi'. The right nostril we relate to the warm sun, and this right side is called the 'pingala nadi'. When the two nadis (channels) are the same temperature, there is no disease in the body. There are some yogic practices which moderate these temperatures.'

The lesson continued as follows:

5. *Suryabhedi Pranayama* helps to heat up the body temperature if you are feeling cold. Close left nostril and inhale through right nostril. Then close both nostrils with thumb and forefinger, and hold breath for as long as is comfortable. Finally breathe out forcefully through left nostril. Repeat conversely and then repeat the whole exercise three times.

6. *Kapalabhati Pranayama* is done by breathing in and out rapidly through the nose while contracting the stomach muscles strongly at each exhalation.

   a. Start by practising a few rounds of Kapalabhati rapid breathing through one nostril with the other closed.

   b. Hold the breath in, lean head back, then forward, then up straight. Breathe out completely through the nose.

   c. Repeat conversely through other nostril.

   d. Repeat exercise with both nostrils together.

These techniques are beneficial for the head, frontal lobes of the brain, sinus and neck.

7. *Loma Viloma Pranayama* (holding the breath out). This should be done only when the student has reached the stage of being able to perform Kapalabhati Pranayama at least twenty rounds with both nostrils together.

   a. After the twenty rounds, breathe out completely, pulling in the stomach muscles (this is called Uddiyana).

   b. Then release the stomach muscles and breathe in, making a 'belly' sound.

This technique is very good for the stomach, circulating oxygen inside the stomach walls. Gastric troubles, acidity, colitis and constipation can be helped by regular practice.

8. *Bhramary Pranayama* (sounding a vocal outbreath). Breathe in through the nose allowing chest to inflate. Hold breath, slightly lowering chin towards chest. Then, while slowly

breathing out, make a smooth outward sound from the throat. This is particularly good for the tonsils.

9. *Kumbhaka Pranayama* (holding the breath in).
    a. Breathe in completely with ease.
    b. Close off the ears with each thumb.
    c. Close the eyes and rest the forefingers on them.
    d. Press the nostrils together with the middle fingers.
    e. Purse the lips and puff out the cheeks.
    f. Holding breath, bend head back, forwards, then hold straight.
    g. Purse the lips again to blast out the held breath completely.

This helps to improve memory, sight, hearing and sense of smell.

10. *Nadishodhan Pranayama* (alternate nostril breathing).
    a. Sit comfortably in a chair or on the floor. Practise alternate nostril breathing by using thumb and forefinger to close each nostril in turn.
    b. Breathe in through one nostril and out slowly through the other.
    c. Repeat for three minutes.
    d. Sit quietly with eyes closed and you will come to feel very comfortable and peaceful in both mind and body, especially chest and abdomen.

The session is always finished with this practice to generate mental peace.

Mr Sharma said, 'I like this restful state, and I can sit for hours and hours feeling at peace with myself and with the world. I mostly use this pranayama with people who have suffered from hypertension and they soon find peace within.'

At the conclusion of the session we thanked Mr Sharma very warmly for all the information and demonstrations he had given us, and took our leave.

Address:
Ram Krishna Vivekananda Yog Ashram, Vishnupuri,
ALIGARH – 202 001.

CHAPTER FIFTEEN

Meeting Dr Swami Gitananda

As I mentioned earlier, after I gave my paper at Kaivalyadhama, I was given a message that Dr Swami Gitananda ('S.G.') would like to have a private talk with me later on. S.G. was reputed to be one of the most eminent international gurus of our time and I was honoured to receive his invitation. That evening Chris and I duly went to his room and met a big, striking, vital man of 77 dressed in a brilliant orange robe. He had copious long silver hair and a silver beard of equal length. He was a most impressive figure.

We sat on his bed and listened, enthralled, to a fascinating story. He told us that it was only a month ago that he had been able to rise up and move about again, after spending twenty months flat on his back as the result of a disastrous accident. It happened when he overbalanced and fell backwards into his swimming-pool sustaining devastating injuries that could never have been foreseen. He fractured his spine and badly damaged his spinal cord in which an infection then developed. Emergency surgery was carried out to remove two blood clots and he then contracted meningitis, which responded in due course to chemotherapy. For more than a year he was completely enclosed in a plaster cast moulded into two pieces so as to cover his entire body from neck to ankles. He was, of course, totally unable to move and for several months he could not even talk. In addition, his hearing and eyesight were seriously impaired.

He told us, 'Yoga has been a way of life for me since the age of twelve, and I can truly say that up until this accident I had never had a day's illness – never a cold, headache, toothache, bowel trouble, or anything of that sort. I feel compensated for my suffering by the fact that, although the accident nearly destroyed me physically, it has given me a new understanding and insight into my patients which I never had before.' In yoga terms he felt that while incapacitated he had become an expert in how to profit from having to remain for more than a year in Shavasana (corpse posture), 'During that time I had plenty of time for introspection and I tuned into the atoms of my body and the Atman (awareness of the indwelling Self). I began to rebuild my inner strength again, and breathed the life back into my body.'

While expressing deep gratitude to all who had cared for him so well, he nevertheless declared, 'Western medicine kept me from dying, but it is yoga that is giving me back my life and health. Other factors which I am sure are contributing to my recovery are the prayers of thousands of my disciples all over the world, and also the fact that I fell in love with my wife all over again – which is the nicest thing that could happen and the best rejuvenator imaginable.'

He took plenty of calcium to promote the regrowth of his damaged bones, and followed a strict vegetarian diet. With the return of some bodily mobility, he began to exercise by stretching his toes, bending his knees, holding objects in his hands, and raising his arms. When, the following year, he was removed from the plaster cast, he was able to sit up in a metal and leather set of belts, gently turning from side to side and lifting his head on a deep inbreath. With the help of a four-legged metal pipe walker he learned how to stand and keep his balance again. He said, 'If I had not really wanted wholeheartedly to walk, and resolved to succeed, I would never have walked again.'

Gradually his battered body began miraculously to regenerate, and his hearing and sight returned. He disciplined himself each month by making a vow for the month ahead: to succeed in feeding himself; to try to get up to a standing position beside his bed; by using ropes instead of the helping hands of others; to climb stairs; to roll over to a prone position, and lift his head and legs to do a modified Bhugana Asana (cobra pose); to swim every day; to crawl like a baby (he maintained that crawling was one of the best exercises possible and should not be left merely to babies.) He exclaimed in heartfelt tones, 'Yoga had always been real to me, but how much more real it became through this shattering experience!'

We were deeply impressed by all he told us. It was S.G.'s unswerving resolve to overcome his injuries, and his dynamic character, together with a rare gift for explaining the most complex aspects of yoga and science in simple everyday terms, that prompted us later to pay a visit to the Ananda Ashram.

Swami Gitananda and the Ananda Ashram

S.G.'s Irish father was a General in the British Army and had accompanied King George V to India before the First World War. He and his Irish Catholic wife remained in India, and later became Hindus. Thus, S.G. was born into the Hindu way of life. At the age of twelve he met and served his guru for many years, until he joined the British Navy at the outbreak of World War Two. He became a Doctor of Surgery and was decorated for his bravery and prowess.

After the war he became a director of the World Health Organisation (WHO), and spent much time in South America. He was a very accomplished heart surgeon, and never lost a patient in 420 operations.

On returning from WHO, he returned to his guru in Pondicherry, at the monastic site of Sri Kambliswami, to continue teaching and disseminating yoga in the tradition of the ancient Rishi of Ashramacharya. His predecessors at this Gurukula Ashram were reputed to have attained phenomenal ages. They lived and taught one of the oldest known cultures, the Dravidian, which includes the Yoga and Saiva Siddhanta tradition of which records go back to 341 BC.

Since 1972, S.G. has rebuilt the ashram around the ancient temple containing relics of the shrine of Kamblis Swami. The new complex is decorated with stone, metal and wooden carvings of the ancient gods and goddesses of Southern India, together with ancient Saiva Siddhantist tombs which are dotted around the lush jungle-like tropical garden. The building, which houses forty or more students, is modern yet retains the spiritual atmosphere of the centuries of Rishi meditation. S.G. arranged for this beautiful and holy place to be listed as a university and registered institution for yoga education. Yoga teachers and medical therapists are trained in indigenous Yoga, Yoga Chikitsa (therapy) and Ayurveda (ancient science of Indian medicine) systems. The courses are at diploma level for beginners and degree level for those already qualified. These qualifications are registered with the Secretary of Education, Pondicherry, the Ministry of Education, and the Ministry of Health in the case of Yoga Chikitsa.

The yoga course covers Prana Chikitsa (breath therapy), Hatha Yoga – asanas, Kriyas, Mudras, Pranayama, yoga relaxation, Jnana Yoga (wisdom of higher knowledge) techniques, and Mantra Yoga (vibration of sound), Kaya Chikitsa (body therapy), paramedical systems, yoga therapy, Mandalas (geometric forms associated with the chakras – psychic vortices of energy), Bindus – the 'mind point' in contact with chakras under the Laya Yoga system (merging with the subtle inner path). All these are overlaid by Ashtanga Yoga, the Royal Path of Yoga covering the dominion of the mind over the body.

The courses take place each year from October to the end of March. Some students may be admitted to other courses taking place parallel to this basic course over a one-month or three-month period. There are also therapeutic yoga treatments carried out from April to September for the benefit of individuals.

When we set off to visit S.G. at his ashram, we began by taking a coach for a 3-hour journey along a dusty bustling track thronged with people who kept boarding the bus regardless of its already being filled to overflowing. At Pondicherry we changed to a scooter rickshaw through the crowded Thattanchavady Industrial Estate, until we eventually arrived at the overwhelming contrast of the haven of peace and splendour that was Ananda Ashram. The gates were opened for us to walk down the path and around a giant circular pool where stood a very high statue of Shiva and Shakti in the Ananda Tandava – the Cosmic Dance.

We were just in time for the evening meal of fruit freshly picked from the garden. Then we attended Satsangha – a fellowship gathering of S.G. with students from India, Italy, Holland and England. Afterwards, S.G. invited us into his room and described the regimen traditionally known as Yoga Sadhana (path of spiritual discipline) based on an old Vedic concept. All the activities were arranged according to the most favourable times for each to have the maximum effect. The day began with meditation from 4 a.m. to 5 a.m. Then followed pranayama from 5 to 6 a.m.; Hatha Yoga from 6 to 8 a.m.; breakfast; instruction in Jnana (disseminative wisdom) kriyas and Raja Yoga kriyas (concentration and relaxation techniques) from 10.30 till noon, followed by a 3½-hour break; Yoga Chikitsa (yoga therapy) is at 3.30 to 5 p.m.; Sanskrit at 5 to 5.30 p.m.; classical mantra chanting at 5.30 to 6 p.m.; a gap of an hour, then Bhajana (devotional song) from 7 to 7.30 p.m.; the evening meditation was at 7.30–8.30 pm; and bedtime was at 10 p.m. S.G. declared that the powerful shakti (energy) generated by the thousands of years of Sadhana on this holy site was available to all students who were prepared to work for it.

After a night's rest, we were interrupted by a loudly clanging gong at 3.45 a.m. which continued for a couple of minutes. We slipped on our yoga clothes, carried a shawl and straw yoga mat, and joined the others in meditation in an upstairs hall. We were kept alert in the stillness of our early morning practice by various insects, tropical birds and tame monkeys which flocked around us. Other noisy contributions were made by the local residents on the industrial estate, who turned up their loud speakers to a

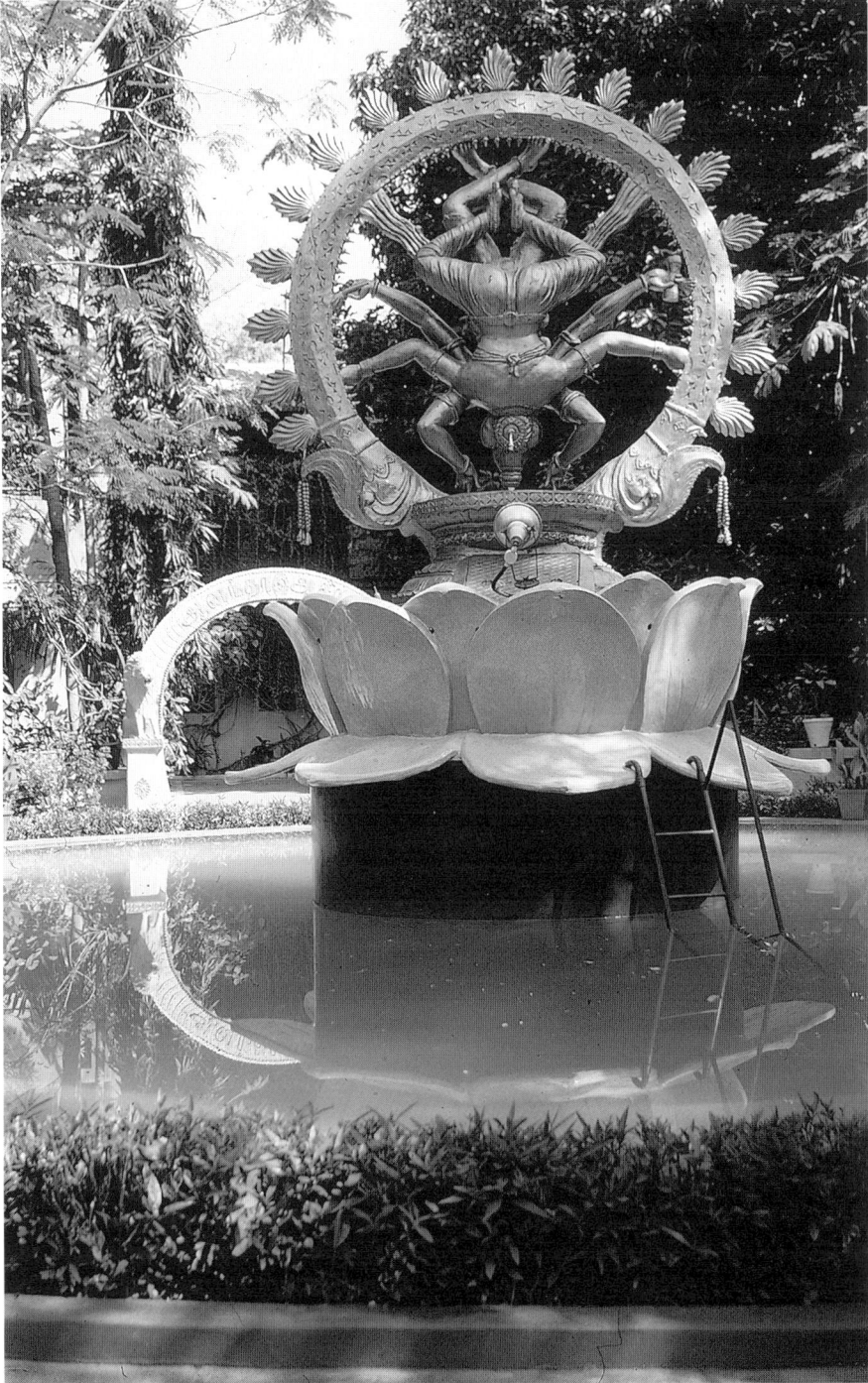

The statue of Shiva and Shakti in the Ananda Tandava – the Cosmic Dance.

deafening pitch, relaying their howling yells and songs. We felt that to overcome these distractions was a real triumph of the spiritual over the material!

After the pranayama session, we climbed up a steep ladder leading to the roof to exercise and sing in greeting to the sun and the activities of the day ahead. Once a week these Hatha Yoga exercises were held on S.G.'s own sandy beach, where we practised Surya Namaskara, saluting the magnificent sunrise as the sun appeared over the sea's horizon.

The early morning exercises were led by S.G's' youthful American wife Meenakshi Devi, while all other theoretical course work was taught by S.G. himself. Their son Ananda, born in 1972 (when S.G. was 72), joined in the yogic way of life, and each day received his academic schooling from Meenakshi who was a graduate in English. She was the editor of 'Yoga Life', an international monthly journal containing practical and philosophical articles on yoga. She had become a naturalised Hindu, and was able to perform the Bharat Natyam (classical Indian dance) beautifully. She organised classes – given by her students – for local children every Sunday, with one teacher dealing with up to 200 children. The children had their lunch in the grounds of the ashram and at the end of the year they were provided with a hand woven ashram yoga uniform.

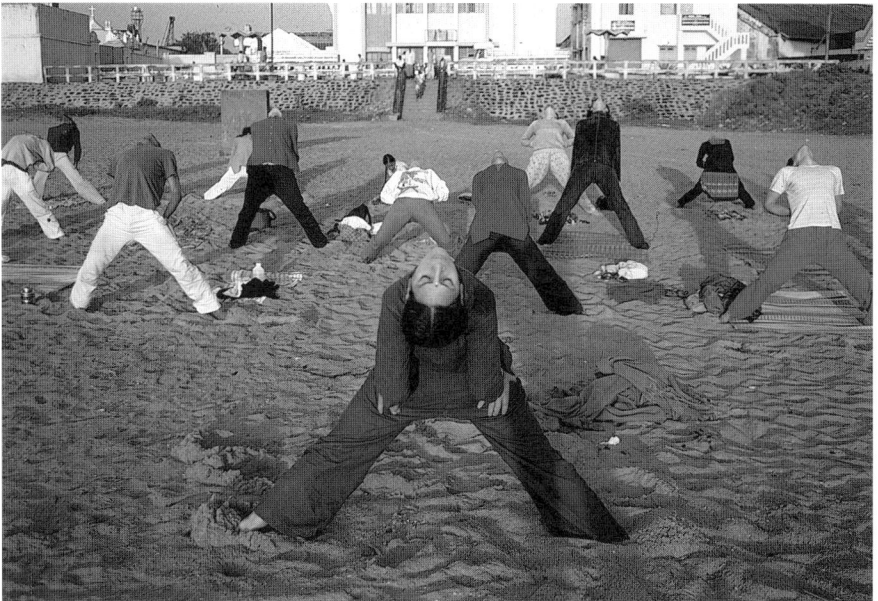

Early morning yoga with Meenakshi on the beach.

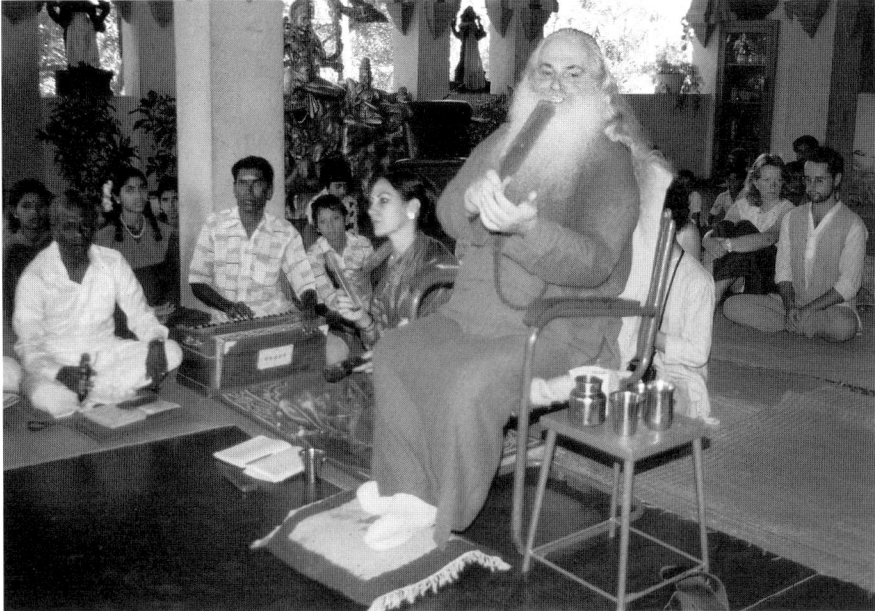

Swami Gitananda leads Bhajana – the singing of devotional songs.

The Ananda Ashram is a full-time haven for people from all walks of life, maintaining Indian culture in its purest form, and counteracting the undesirable pressures and stresses of life in the world outside.

S.G. told us, 'Meenakshi is involved with more than 1,000 children here, and fortunately in India they don't suffer from problems like rickets, bone deformation, etc., because of their natural lifestyle. You won't find a hole in their teeth, they never need dental care. There may be a few who are disabled, but we don't treat them any different from the others.' 'Modern educationalists could take a leaf out of S.G.'s book when it comes to promoting the integration of all children.

'During the last twenty years or so, yoga education has been placed by various governments under the unfavourable classification of 'Physical Education and Sport.' By limiting and categorising yoga in this mechanical way, 'teaching from without', so to speak, instead of teaching from within, much of its richness in energising the inner human potential and drawing on spiritual resources has been lost.

'We estimate that 10,000 children and young persons have learned something about yoga in the last ten years from our programme. Some have just heard the word 'yoga' and gained a vague idea of its meaning, before negative forces have dragged them away. Others have developed to some extent, before dropping out for this or that reason. A few have managed to make it through the ten years, and shine like stars in their own environment, and are lights to those with whom they associate. Why can't more ashrams and yoga centres in India and around the world conduct programmes similar to this one, reaching out to the children in their community? Perhaps a whole new generation could arise capable of realising their full potential through yoga!'

I asked S.G. how he envisaged yoga therapists using their certificates. He replied, 'The yoga therapist is ahead of his time, in that the West has never thought of yoga as wholism. Therefore it will take time for the therapists to find a sphere in which they can function. We suggest to the youngsters that they should first qualify as medical practitioners, physiotherapists, or even masseurs, and should then begin to incorporate yoga practices into their work. Their superiors are bound to see that yoga is complementary to western therapies, and in time the demand for similar training will arise.

'The trainees are encouraged to embark upon the yogic path in a step-by-step correspondence course dealing with philosophy, psychology, hygiene and diet, and instruction in pranayama and basic diet. Although the written word is never a satisfactory substitute for personal contact with a guru, there are not many who can afford the necessary time and expense of learning from the guru direct or living in his ashram. Our Study Pack gives fifty two lessons into what classical yoga is all about, and provides suitable practices to prepare the sincere student for the higher and more complex phases of yoga which can only be taught by a guru.' S.G. explained that until recently yoga had to a large extent been denied to the general Indian community because most ashrams were financed by elite members of society who were spiritually inclined. Therefore, he said, the ashrams had been failing in their duty to the community, but the situation had now improved to some extent. I asked for his views on the extent to which disabled people in India could benefit from yoga, and he replied that benefit was assured because of the wonderful power of yoga to evoke from the body its own natural powers of healing at almost any level.

He stated, 'The political side also comes into the picture. The Indian government has not utilised Indian indigenous medicine as it should – there should be a Yoga Chikitsa expert in every state. You will find Coca Cola caps and bottles, empty packets of cigarettes, and empty bottles of alcohol in the smallest and most remote villages, but no medical services, let alone yoga. People say to us, 'Why don't you yogis do more?' but we cannot fill the gap on our own. There should be a coordinated project, otherwise it is just left to isolated institutions like Ananda Ashram to do what we can. We give 6 months' training to medical therapists and yoga teachers, and during the remaining 6 months we operate a clinic for outpatients most of whom are sufferers the doctors have given up. I welcome trainees who are doctors and nurses, because if we can show them that yoga works for them, they will certainly spread the good work in their own practices. Occasionally the doctors may send me a patient whom they would not touch with a 10-foot pole, yet they expect me to work with this patient, using Yoga Chikitsa, on a one-to-one basis – which is simply not practicable. These problems ought to be solved, so far as possible, by prevention rather than cure. In order to accomplish this, we will have to change the present social order; train more qualified Yoga Chikitsa practitioners, and move towards a less spiritual form of yoga which is more community-orientated for the general health of the people. In that way we can take on a new role in society.

'Medical science today is uneasy about its methods, realising that in some cases its results are very poor. I am sure that if science and yoga could be brought together to work in concert, the number of mental patients would greatly decrease, proving that yoga is a much more satisfactory form of treatment for this problem.'

S.G. acknowledged that the West had useful technology to offer, but said that they should seize the opportunity to investigate yoga therapy. Unfortunately they did not know what they should be researching or where to start. 'I feel that western science is losing its bearings and its purpose, it is soulless and has no philosophy, and yoga could supply that need. The West has materialistic science, we in India have the concept of soul and there could be a beautiful blending of the two, to everyone's advantage.'

Swami Gitananda died on 29 December 1993 at the age of 88 and his wife Meenakshi Devi and son Ananda have continued teaching yoga at the Ananda Ashram in the tradition of Ashtanga Rishi Culture Yoga.

Recommended reading: *Yoga Step-By-Step*, a fifty-two lesson training course in the ancient art and science of classical yoga.

Address:
Ananda Ashram, Thattanchavady, PONDICHERRY – 605 009.

CHAPTER SIXTEEN

Visit to Jalawral Institute of Post-Graduate Medical Education Research (JIPMER)

S.G. took us to visit his local hospital. We arrived at the Jalawral Institute of Post-Graduate Medical Education (JIPMER), a huge prestigious institute training doctors from all over the world in all forms of medical research and treatment. Swamiji was warmly welcomed by the hospital staff who regarded him as 'a miracle of a yogi, standing so straight and looking so well' after such an ordeal of paralysis and disability.

S.G. was eager to introduce us to Dr Modan Mohan of Srinagar, Kashmir, an eminent physiologist and lecturer in the physiology department. Prior to S.G.'s accident, Dr Mohan had collaborated with him on an in-depth study of yoga and they had jointly published a number of papers on yoga for both healthy and sick

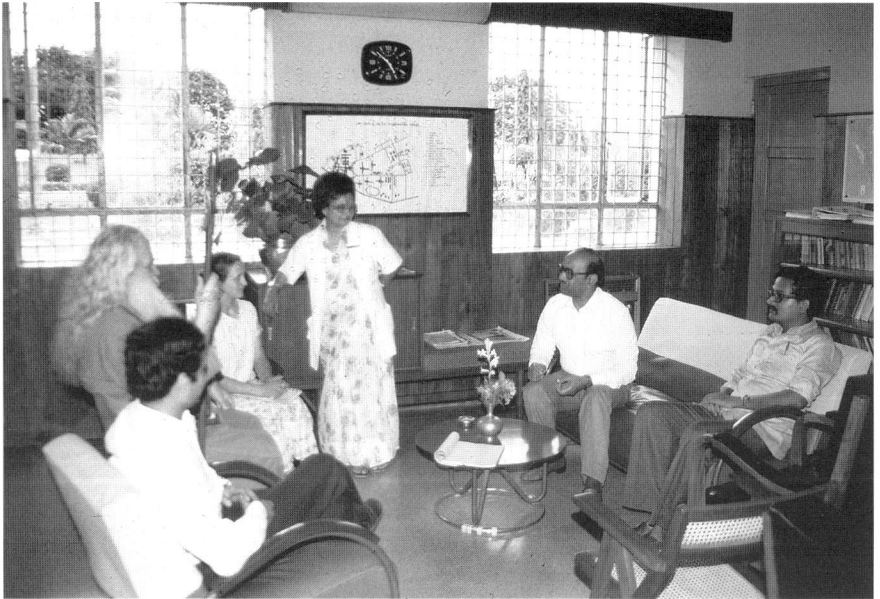

S.G. arranged a meeting for me with the Principal of JIPMER and some Heads of Department.

people. Dr Mohan had originally received basic tuition in yoga from S.G. and he practised asanas and pranayamas daily. He gave S.G. his complete cooperation, along with his team in the department of physiology, to establish the value of yoga techniques, particularly Savitri Pranayama (rhythmical breath) and Shavasana (relaxation in corpse posture). Through these practices, together with meditation, there was a remarkable reduction in oxygen consumption to bring about complete relaxation of mind and body. Since these techniques are not difficult to perform, and, unlike drugs, do not involve any side-effects, it would seem sensible to carry out more studies on their value in stress-induced disorders and other illnesses.

Dr Mohan handed me their scientific paper on 'Cardiorespiratory Changes during Savitri Pranayama and Shavasana,' in which S.G. wrote:

'Savitri Pranayama, the Rhythmic Breath, is one of the important pranayamas taught at Ananda Ashram, particularly for the valuable relaxation it affords if used for 10–20 minutes at a single practice. Savitri Pranayama is also known to produce an outstanding change in the metabolism of the yoga practitioner, deliberately reducing the respiratory rate to just over $2\frac{1}{2}$ breaths per minute ($8 \times 4 \times 8 \times 4$). The heart rate also falls to a very low level and a hypometabolic state is observed. The practice is neurologically parasympatholytic and has been known to reduce oxygen consumption drastically, thus indicating deep relaxation of the practitioner. Many yogis practice an even slower rate of $16 \times 8 \times 16 \times 8$, or a single breath in the period of a minute. My Guru, Swami Kanakananda Bhrigu, taught me that twenty minutes of Savitri Pranayama is equal to eight hours of anabolic (healthy) sleep. The recent tests at JIPMER indicate that the actual value of twenty minutes of this Savitri Pranayama is equal to two full nights of restful sleep. The meditation used in this controlled experiment was simply to 'watch the breath' in its rhythmic pattern for two to five minutes, then transfer the concentration point of the established rhythm to a point between the tip of the nose and upper lip, a concentration point in Pranayama Kosha. This is also referred to as Shanti Pranayama in this form.'

Dr Mohan took us round his laboratory to see the research equipment used to measure the body's biological and metabolic functions while practising yoga. S.G. supplied the yoga practitioners and tests showed that yogis can control their breathing and heartbeat. The tests proved that persons trained in Savitri Pranayama were saving as much as 27 per cent of their blood-oxygen, whereas others tested who did not practise these techniques were using up all their blood-oxygen, with consequent susceptibility to fatigue. Tests done with a spirometer showed that some patients exhaled all the oxygen they had inhaled, which was a handicap since when they breathed in, the air was not circulating properly to nourish the cellular body.

The equipment used to test the body at rest was also used to check out certain diseases of the lungs by observing how the patient was breathing, and for example determining whether or not the air sacs were accepting the oxygen. In fact scientific equipment used in hospitals can detect a number of problems which could be prevented by the use of yoga.

The equipment used to test the body in activity was a bicycle wired up with electrodes from the handlebars to the laboratory apparatus. The subject was put through standard tests – whilst they were performing various movements the effects of, for example, the basal metabolism (the energy changes such as the beating of the heart, respiration, body temperature etc.) were monitored. Various comparative tests were carried out to test the patient's stamina. These were standard tests on the bicycle, followed by six minutes of yoga, followed in turn by more cycle practice. Six months later the procedure was repeated. It was found that patients who had practised yoga regularly during the intervening period had increased their powers of physical endurance on the cycle.

The electrical processing tests showed the long fibres of muscles contracting with the electromagnetic responses, causing hardening of the muscles. This was not the direct result of the exercises done, but was a more complicated chain of causation. The tests proved that muscular reactions under the electromagnetic stimulus varied in individuals and could be used to indicate psychosomatic symptoms treatable by yoga.

S.G. showed us the 'Polygraph 7' which monitored the brain for tumours, abscesses, scar tissue, blood clots, etc. This machine was also useful for testing electrical, magnetic and neurological fields in the brain under the influence of pranayama. S.G. also used it to test his students when meditating, to find out if they were successfully producing alpha waves (the initial stage of meditation).

Dr Bhargava, the Principal of JIPMER, sent a message asking S.G. to call on him in his office and invited us to accompany him. Dr Bhargava was delighted to see Swamiji miraculously on his feet again and also expressed great interest in my experiences in yoga with people with learning disabilities. He told me that they had recently built a gigantic Rehabilitation Unit in the hospital complex to treat people from all over India who had severe difficulty in looking after themselves. Unfortunately, in this top western-standard medical institution work on the Rehabilitation Unit had to be halted because they had run out of funds for equipment and staff. Subsequently he realised the potential of having yoga teaching in this unit when it could afford to open. He asked us if we could come back later for a meeting with other Heads of Department to discuss the project.

This we did four days later, and met Dr Moharty (Orthopaedic Department) Dr (Mrs) Trivedy (Psychiatric Department) and Dr Madan Mohan (Physiology Department). The meeting lasted two hours, during which great interest was shown in my yoga programmes back in England. There were, however, mixed feelings about introducing yoga into the eventual rehabilitation curriculum. Dr Trivedy was hesitant because she wondered whether the discipline for practice might not interfere with the hospital's established routine. The Ananda Ashram was almost next door to the hospital, and S.G. was eager to offer yoga teachers trained in Yoga Chikitsa along with the necessary equipment, which after all consisted only of yoga mats. He urged that yoga should be introduced into the new unit right from the start.

The Principal then expressed his views. He said he had made up his mind that yoga should be introduced for disabled people as soon as the unit opened. He said that the hospital already funded an acupuncturist and that a yoga therapist could be financed through the same channel. He thought that some members of the hospital staff might be interested to learn yoga for the benefit of themselves and their patients.

S.G. said, 'The problem here is, I can supply the yoga therapists, but they are not medical graduates, so there is going to be some bias. At the moment there isn't a system to study both, but in time the demand will be there. So gradually we intend to mushroom the number of trained yoga therapists, even though in the early stages we will be creating these workers ahead of their time, so to speak.'

A few months later I was very pleased to hear that a yoga programme led by S.G.'s trained yoga teachers was under way at JIPMER with 168 doctors and nurses. I am confident that the introduction of yoga into reputable hospitals such as JIPMER will give new confidence to disabled people and will gain them social acceptance in the outside world.

While at Ananda Ashram, we saw many cases of marked improvement in physical disability, the most striking of which was Sushi Bhattacharya. He was a young man from West Bengal who was working at the ashram as S.G.'s right hand. He was aged twenty-four and had been four times Gold Medallist yoga champion of Tamil Nadu. We were fortunate that he gave us a demonstration that we were able to video. He performed seemingly miraculous contortions showing complete mastery of Hatha Yoga through total control of mind and body.

It transpired that at the age of eighteen he had suffered from a number of serious diseases. Not finding any help from ordinary medicine, he turned to yoga as a last resort and learned the natural way to a permanent and total cure. In a single year, the remarkable improvement in his health enabled him to enter and win the yoga championship for his State, competing against about 650 other entrants. His success on three subsequent occasions, and the magnificent performance we witnessed, convinced us that he would be able to defend his title for a long time to come!

Address:

JIPMER (Jawaharlal Institute of Postgraduate Medical Education and Research), Dhanvantari Nagar, PONDICHERRY – 605 006.

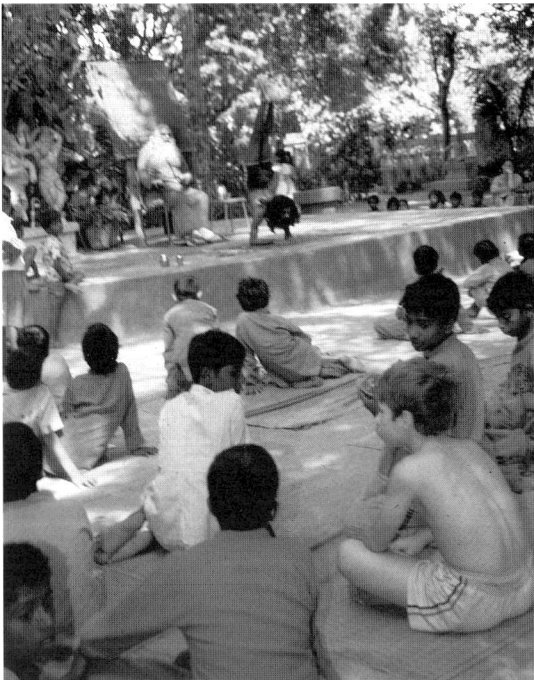

Sushi Bhattacharya's demonstration in front of Swami Gitananda.

CHAPTER SEVENTEEN

Report on the YOCOCEN
'Yoga–Nature–Ahimsa' Conference

Conference of YOCOCEN (International Yoga Coordination
Centre) held at Bhartiya Vidya Bhawan, New Delhi
December 1984. Organised by Dr C. P. Mehra.

Written by Christopher and Maria Gunstone

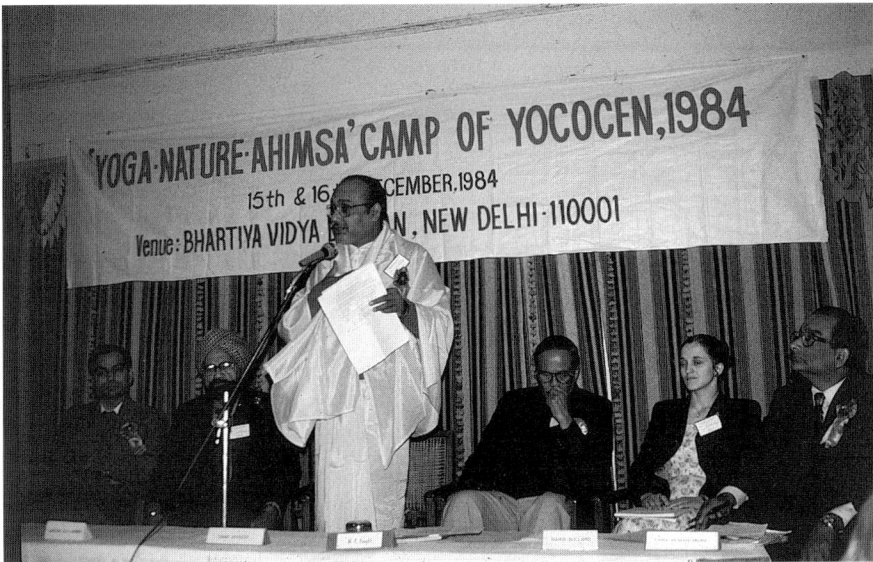

*Non-violence is the meaning of 'Ahimsa' and this conference covered
the subject of peace ...*

The first speaker, Swami P. Saraswata, Director of two hundred
yoga organisations in USA, took a critical line, demanding 'In five
thousand years, what has yoga done for India? Why are 80 per
cent of the population still poor and ignorant? What has God done
for the people? Is God responsible for the Suffering? Why are
there still political and social problems between Hindus, Moslems,
Sikhs, when yoga means union? Take a look at our yoga attitudes
and customs. There is a radical division between all religions, and
this is quite wrong. Even when yoga is taught in schools, outside

of the yogic state of peace, violence and separation are still encountered. Why fool ourselves by saying that our country is the best? We must analyse ourselves to find out what is going wrong. Our troubles are not always due to individual karma (the universal law of cause and effect) or fate. The truths set out in old books are great, but we must be pragmatic and keep up with the times.' He concluded by saying 'The middle path is best, to combine old and new ideas.'

Shri Mool Raj Anand, naturopath, expounded his 'Tragedies of the Human Race', as ignorant and misguided man sought to improve on God's work. There were so many divergences and contradictions between beliefs and intentions, and actual performance. Shri Mool maintained that the basic cause of man's misery was inflammation caused by meat-eating, cooked foods, too much sugar and salt, and drugs. He told us that at the age of 61 he had not even been able to climb stairs, but he then changed his lifestyle, and now, twenty years later at the age of 81, he worked a 16-hour day without fatigue. He stated that the body was self-sufficient and self-directing, and it produced fevers as a cleansing process to get rid of toxins. Fasting acted as a cure. A benevolent energy was working in everyone to repair cells that wore out and bad food interfered with this process.

He spoke about 'Omni' – all knowledge beyond the senses and the wonderful creation of the Almighty whose wisdom and power could maintain everything it created. The flowers which filled the air with fragrance were an example of beneficent creation in manifestation, as opposed to the person who committed a vindictive crime motivated by destructive emotions like hatred and revenge. Shri Mool suggested that everyone should be educated as to what to put into their bodies. He also mentioned that they should question whether they really needed to kill beautiful animals and commit them to flames in order to make a meal. This would be a good start in improving the 'inner personality of man'. Then, people would give thought to the welfare of other creatures that shared our planet and not wish to harm them in any way. One of the aims of Ahimsa awareness was to educate everyone in the value of Sattvic (pure) foods for health and well-being. Foods like fruit and vegetables, which were cheap, plentiful and harmless, should be chosen, thus removing the darkness of ignorance, tragedy and ill-health, and avoiding violence.

Shri H. Sharma, Adviser to the Indian Education Department, spoke of yoga's acceptance in the curricula of some schools, though sometimes it was wrongly labelled 'Physical Education'. PE was in fact a completely different subject of competitive exercise for the strong, whereas the strength of yoga lay in self-control and harmonious relationships. Why had non-violence reached a high point in India and not the rest of the world? Shri Sharma's friend Mahatma Gandhi had influenced India because he went to the lowest among the people and lifted them up. The Gandhi film gained worldwide popularity because it dedicated in practical and vivid terms Gandhi's powerful message of non-violence which in the end achieved its aim.

Shri K. C. Tuli, Lecturer in Psychology, Zakir Hussain College, Delhi, gave a talk on 'Modern Life, Stress and Yoga'. He referred to the modern media's unbalanced reporting of constant bad news from all over the world, which perpetuated a climate of fear and tension, and aggravated stress which had never been so intense as it was today. He suggested yoga as being 'the safe way out', and emphasised that now was an appropriate juncture to recognise and cultivate a system of philosophy and practice which emerged from the ancient civilisation of India to produce a solution to the problems which beset twentieth-century man all over the world. Yoga consisted of a tremendous body of knowledge which was as perfect in its way as any of the sciences like physics or chemistry. It was a rich abundant knowledge which could be a panacea for the problems of modern man, and which also had the potential for bringing about perfection. The science of yoga provided the perfect style of living which everyone of us should endeavour to incorporate in our lives, and thus express the perfection of God and infinite universe.

Dr C. P. Mehra, Trustee and Hon. Secretary-General of YOCOCEN, gave a demonstration of therapeutic Hastha Mudras, which were movements and gestures performed by joining or bending hands, fingers, wrists and arms. He said that the sages used these to control disease and keep the body fit for the pursuit of spiritual upliftment and self-realisation. The practice of Hastha Mudras kept the glands functioning in a healthy state. Performing the mudras during meditation, together with japa (rhythmic recitations), bhajans (ceremonial songs), and other religious rites, had a beneficial effect on the physical, nervous and mental health of the performer.

Dr Mehra also gave lectures on 'Strategies for Social Transformation and on Self-realisation', and on Kundalini (arousal of psychic subtle energy). In the latter he said, 'Scientists have so far failed to measure Kundalini, and cannot do so without becoming Sadhakas (disciples), disciplining themselves for 3–6 months and undergoing the yogic experience.' He emphasised that the process of Kundalini arousal normally took years.

Pandit Shambhu Nath lectured on 'The Psychosomatic approach to Yoga' with special reference to Patanjali's system of yoga discipline on the eightfold path, compiled in the second century BC.

Mr M. P. Pandit, from Sri Aurobindo's ashram, Pondicherry, made some valuable comments on Kundalini Sadhana (discipline) and conducted a meditation class. He also spoke about Yoga-Union and said that there was a great deal of disagreement among gurus regarding their own particular yoga techniques, which unfortunately had the effect of keeping yoga from the people. 'You cannot shut up God in one system, to the exclusion of another. With the explosion of twentieth-century knowledge, yoga must be available to all. Elitism has no place in this, because there is no one way to serve God.'

During the questions and answers period, a very heated debate took place. The conclusion reached was that no one part of yoga was wrong in relation to another – it was all part of an eightfold path, which was Yoga-Union and which therefore must be open to accept new ways of reaching the goal.

Swami Akhileshji said that Yoga Ahimsa excluded everything that disturbed the mind. Man must make peace with himself and with society. Peace was the result of yoga practice. He maintained that if we removed pollution from our environment, then there would be Ahimsa. He said there were three things to develop in one's life: knowledge, character and good work.

The validation was delivered by Shri H. Kumar Kaul, Director of Patanjali Yoga Institute and Principal of S.D. College, Barhala, Punjab. He taught English at the College, and also over the past few years had been conducting Hatha Yoga sessions daily from 6 to 7 a.m. for students and non-students, with considerable success.

At his college there were approximately 4,000 students who received formal education, and of these 120 chose to attend the early morning yoga sessions.

Shri Kumar Kaul said, 'Young people have lost their bearings and lost control of their own destiny under the impact of science, technology and democracy. They have become antisocial. Education becomes a farce if it deviates from character-formation and reform from within oneself. Our health has been damaged by extensive pollution of air, water, and soil through the use of pesticides and toxins. The tragedy of Bhopal is still vivid in our minds. People may be called 'civilised' now, but are they really happy? Why do they need pills to sleep, laxatives for their bowels, aspirins for their aching heads? Lust for money has corrupted their hearts. It is better not to reject scientific achievement outright, but to re-orientate machines towards stable equilibrium with nature and not against it. The solution to man's physical ailments, psychological maladies, and emotional tensions lies with yoga, which is the most practical preventive and curative remedy to meet the demands of modern life. If you wish to change society, you must first change yourself. My students ask me, 'How do breathing exercises extend the family budget?' Everything is interrelated. Through yoga man makes friends with himself and with nature. Man cannot remain idle, but work is not everything; the key is the attitude in which he performs it.'

The conference did not come up with any precise plans to solve India's and humanity's problems. The consensus was, that, man having been thrust into the twentieth century, with all his failures and successes, to make his own way in life, therefore it was up to individuals to get to grips with changing themselves as well as society. Being a yogi did not mean cutting oneself off from the rest of humanity. To combine yoga with politics worked in the best interests of society, as Mahatma Gandhi successfully demonstrated.

A number of practical demonstrations were given during the course of the conference, which we were allowed to video. These consisted of:

1. Shankh Mad – sounding of conch shell, the purpose of which was only explained in Hindi, but we gathered that it was designed to focus the mind and spirit on what was to follow. It was performed by Shesh Pal Rastog of the Academy of Yoga.

2. Vastra Dhanti – swallowing and extracting 7-metres of muslin cloth, which cleanses the walls of the oesophagus and stomach. Performed by Shri Anshu Tiwari.

3. Sutra Neti – passing a rubber tube up each nostril in turn and out through the mouth. This cleanses the nasal passages.

4. Jala Neti – pouring salt water through one nostril and out of the other to clear nasal congestion. Performed by Shri S. I. Khanna, editor of 'Saral Yog', a quarterly yoga magazine.

5. Drinking milk through the nose to purify the nasal cavities. Performed by Shri Ajit Mehra.

6. A spinal massage given by Shri N. V. Kulkarni.

7. Hatha Yoga sessions (physical postures) conducted by Yoga-charya Shri Ramantar Sharma and Kumari Bharati of the Aligarh Muslim University.

8. Further Hatha Yoga asanas with Pranayama (breathing techniques to control life force), directed by Smt.Shanta Dhinga, to relieve any pain.

9. Jeevan Tatava Sadhana – development of life force, performed by Shri S. L. Khanna.

In Shri S. L. Khanna's talk and demonstration on the development of the life force, an assistant demonstrated the postures in accordance with Shri Khanna's instructions, as shown below. Each asana was completed by the assistant resting while taking three breaths. When breathing in, he was told to make the vibration of 'OM' in his mind, and when breathing out to send the 'OM' vibration away from the body in imagination. This enabled the mind to become free of the body and gain refreshment on higher planes.

Rotation of Shoulders – (Sakand Chalan).

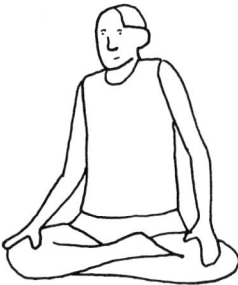

Rotate one shoulder at a time for 35 rotations, forward and then backward. Finish by relaxing with three 'OM' breaths.

Benefits: Removes any congestion in chest and shoulders. It has good effect on liver, spleen and eyes. It helps ease spondylosis. Thyroid and parathyroid glands are rejuvenated.

Rolling of the Navel – (Nabhi Chalan).

While lying supine, place palms on the ground and feet together. Roll on to your left and right side alternately, in such a way that your head remains unturned. Roll 55 times each side. Relax with three 'OM' breaths.

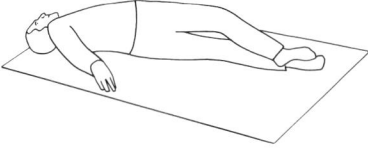

Benefits: This is the best exercise to remove indigestion. It kindles the fire of appetite (Vrik Agni). The idea was taken from a crocodile, who swallows his food and rolls on sand for digestion. It helps cure gaseous trouble.

Thigh Expansion – (Antar Chalan).

Place the right heel on top of the left knee. Lower the right knee and thigh on right side, so that the right knee touches the ground. Retain for 20 seconds, then lift up the knee into first position. Practise for three times. Repeat with left leg three times. Relax with three 'OM' breaths.

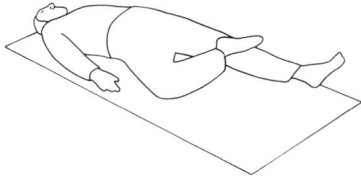

Benefits: It removes constipation. Liver, spleen and intestines are stimulated.

Child Persistence – (Bal Machlan).

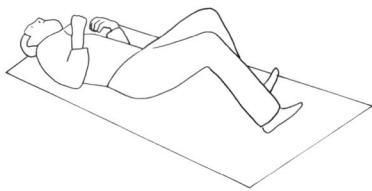

Shri Khanna ended the session by telling his assistant to shake himself all over and then laugh really loudly for a while, visualising himself as a child feeling healthy, bright and lively.

Benefits: This exercise rejuvenates both mind and body.

Relaxation (Shavasana).

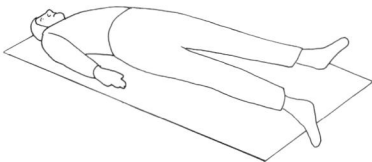

Lying flat on ground relaxing with three 'OM' breaths.

CHAPTER EIGHTEEN

Yogacharya S. Janikiraman

I was referred to Janikiraman by Robert Hughes of Hartfield House Yoga Centre, London. Robert had taught yoga in a psychiatric hospital for more than ten years, and he was my prime inspiration in applying the power of yoga to people's special needs. He told me that Janikiraman was a kind good man from whom he had learnt much valuable information about yoga.

Janikiraman lived in Bangalore, and was Honorary Director of Atma Jyothi, which means divine spark in every human being. Janikiraman welcomed us warmly in his non-residential centre for yoga therapy and spiritual activities. He took his time getting to know us. We exchanged life experiences and he told us a good deal about himself and provided much material concerning his activities, various forms of yoga, and techniques of yoga therapy.

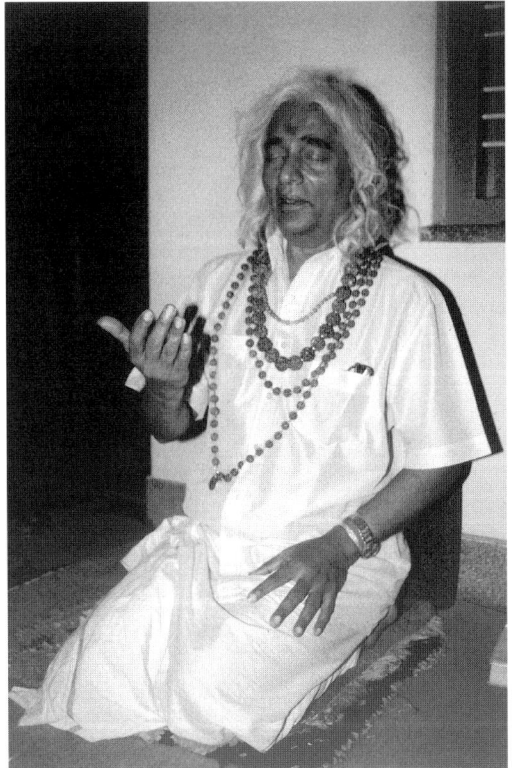

Yogacharya Janikiraman.

Janikiraman was born in 1922, fortunately into a yoga family. As a child he learnt from his father how to worship through devotional song and when he sang to Chris and myself he became like a child enraptured with the love of life. He had received darshan (insight into the laws of the universe and union with God), as well as being blessed by many saints including Swami Sivananda. He had studied Tantra Shastra (the sacred scriptures of ceremonial rites) and yoga with Swami Gitananda, and was devotee of Sai Baba, the modern avatar of India. He had a BSc. (Hons) degree and had been Chief Quality Control Inspector for Hindustan Aeronautics. During that stage of his life, he divided his time between his work, his family and healing. He demonstrated and lectured on yoga from a sound scientific and medical point of view for the cure of disease and rehabilitation of sufferers both in India and in different parts of the world.

In 1978 he compiled a comprehensive booklet 'Practical Yoga Therapy' based on his system of a very practical, gentle and sensible kind applied to hundreds of patients and also doctors of the allopathic, ayurvedic and homeopathic disciplines. All of them benefited in improved health for themselves and their friends and patients to whom they recommended the techniques.

At the age of sixty, Janikiraman retired from this aeronautical post in order to devote himself to Sadhana (Path of Spiritual Discipline). It was at this stage that we visited and underwent thirteen days of intensive study with him. He described his knowledge in terms of twentieth-century technology; for instance he said, 'When we want an engine as good as the Rolls Royce we contact the experts to supply us with the engine's system. In the same way, when studying yoga you have to start from where the ancient rishis (seers) formulated the system of yoga that leads one to a new vision and realisation in the context of today's society.'

I discovered that Janakiraman shared with me a common misfortune, in that he too had broken his neck some years back. He maintained that his prayer and yoga practices had helped to restore his neck to normal. Even so, he stressed that asanas which put pressure on the neck should be avoided, in particular the Neck and Head Balance (Sarvangasana and Sirshasana). He said, 'There is no reason to gamble and irritate the neck by doing those exercises, when there are so many other exercises to benefit from without risk.'

Janakiraman's main activity nowadays was spreading the message of universal love and healing through the traditional forms of yoga which had held sway for thousands of years. He said that the ancient seers required their disciples, who came in search of self-realisation through yoga, to follow a code of behaviour: Patanjali's – 'steps in yoga for the householder' (the eightfold path). These were as follows :

1. Yamas. There are five yamas of self-restraint: non-violence, truthfulness, non-stealing, continence and non-covetousness.

2. Niyamas. There are five niyamas of religious observance: purity, contentment, austerity study and surrender to God.

   These two together constitute codes of conduct which are similar to the Ten Commandments of the western Bible, governing thought, word, and deed.

3. Asanas – postures. The teachers of old had noted how wild animals were in complete harmony with their natural environment and these masters took certain positions in which the animals sat, moved and slept, and adapted them into asanas and Kriyas – cleansing techniques. These were a series of postures and movements which they found through experiment could stabilise and direct the energy of the body.

4. Pranayamas – breath control. The masters similarly developed a system of breathing exercises which controlled and directed the vital force of both body and mind.

   There were many eager young disciples, full of impetuousness and zeal, who were too impatient just to sit still and relax as a preliminary to working towards their goal. By constant practise of asanas and pranayamas and incorporating the yamas and niyamas into their daily lives, the disciples were able to develop the control and stability necessary for spiritual development. Moreover it was discovered that the asanas and pranayamas had a curative effect on physical and mental disorders, not only making an ailing body healthy, but also making a healthy body healthier. In this way, yoga therapy was born and each asana and pranayama was found to benefit particular diseases.

5. Pratyahara – sense withdrawal.

6. Dharana – concentration.

7. Dhyana – meditation.

8. Samadhi – merger with the Divine.

Janakiraman said, 'The desire for God-realisation was the original cause of yoga, and the achievement of the desire was the effect. If the cause is forever pursued, the effect will take care of itself. If someone lies, cheats, or indulges in sensual pleasures, no amount of asanas and pranayamas will evoke the illimitable power of yoga, but a good deal of evil can be got rid of if we are able to control the subtler levels of being. It is no use polishing the outside if there is nothing inside. We have to learn to detach ourselves in order to earn the supreme reward of joy, and this is done by withdrawing the senses and being at one with the Universal Soul. Man's mind is part of the Universal Mind and is connected to every other mind. Yoga has discovered the laws that develop the personality and the soul.'

Address:
Yogachara S. Janikiraman, Atma Jyoti, 297, 10th Main Street,
3rd Block, Jayanagar, BANGALORE – 560 011.

CHAPTER NINETEEN

Spina Bifida – a success story

For over six years, Janikiraman had been prescribing yoga therapy for a child born with spina bifida. He arranged for this
child's mother, Mrs S. Prahala, to bring the child to meet me at
his ashram. This turned out to be a moving story. To give a clear
picture, the following is a report jointly written by Mr and Mrs
Prahala about their daughter:

Our spina bifida baby Amba was born in June 1978 in Delhi.
She had a 2-inch diameter myelocoele (protrusion of the spinal
cord through a defect in a vertebra) in the lumbo-sacral region
at her birth. Within a few hours she was examined by the specialist of the All India Institute of Medical Sciences, and we were
told that it was a hopeless case; the child would not only have
no control over her limbs, but would also suffer from incontinence
of the bladder and bowels. It was also usual for the brain to
suffer some damage, and therefore Amba would probably be
mentally disabled. Thus, unable to walk and confined to a wheelchair, having no control over her bladder and bowels, perhaps
with learning disabilities, she would lead a vegetable existence.
The doctors therefore refused to close the spine, and told us that
the best thing to do was to 'let nature take its course'. In any
case observation for at least six months would be necessary before
any surgery could be contemplated.

We were naturally alarmed, not knowing anything about spina
bifida. We began making inquiries, and also looked through some
books, which only reinforced what the doctors had said. Amba's
condition fulfilled two of the criteria laid down by Dr Lorber,
namely the spina bifida was on the lower half of the spine, and
her legs seemed to be paralysed. We resigned ourselves to our fate.

When Amba was two weeks old she was brought home from
the nursing home where she was born. We started simple
physiotherapy in the shape of straightening and massaging her
legs. The wound on her spine was dressed regularly to avoid any
risk of infection. We noticed that she could stay dry for about
two to three hours, and we were told that possibly her incontinence was not of the worst type.

About three weeks after her birth, we noticed small movements in her legs, and since no such movement was expected on the basis of what the doctors had told us, we were pleasantly surprised. We consulted the doctors again, and they advised closure of the spine. When a torch was shone through the myelocoele, it was sufficiently 'transparent' to encourage the doctor to think that closure of the spine was worthwhile.

This was done when Amba was one month old. She stood up to the operation well, though we were worried about her high temperature a few days after the operation. Great care was taken to reduce the danger of infection, and the wound on her spine was dressed only in an operating theatre until it healed.

Amba was brought to Bangalore when she was two months old. We consulted our paediatrician, and also an orthopaedic surgeon. The paediatrician was frankly aghast that we had had the spine closed, and warned us that in 95 per cent of such cases hydrocephalus (water on the brain) would develop and there would be damage to the brain. We were therefore asked to measure the circumference of the head at regular intervals, and also to look out for any signs of the onset of hydrocephalus such as vomiting, fever, etc. The orthopaedic surgeon, however, was not so pessimistic. After studying the X-rays, he advised use of a heavily padded napkin to keep the legs apart, and also prescribed daily physiotherapy for the hips, knees and ankles.

We noticed enlargement of the head within two months of the closure of the spine. The paediatrician felt that there was no immediate worry, and the situation should be watched in case the hydrocephalus arrested itself and no surgical intervention was necessary.

About this time we met Yogacharya Janikiraman, who was engaged in the study of the therapeutic aspects of yoga, and he recommended a couple of exercises, and also the intoning of the word 'OM' by the mother with her hand on the child's fontenelle (located at the top of the head). We found that this seemed to relax the fontenelle, as if some vital energy flowed from the mother to the child.

When Amba was six months old the enlargement of the head was clearly noticeable, and we were beginning to get worried. There was no vomiting or any other manifestation of severe pressure on the brain such as the 'sunset sign' in the eyes. Her general progress was quite satisfactory, and when she was eight months old she began to speak a few words. After a debate lasting nearly three months it was decided to insert a shunt (pudenz valve) to relieve the pressure on Amba's brain. This was duly performed, and so far (thankfully) no revision of the shunt has been found necessary. Incidentally, just before her shunting Amba was able to pull herself up to a sitting position from a reclining position, in spite of the heaviness of her head.

The shunt was an immediate success, in that Amba's development progressed rapidly thereafter. At about a year, however, she developed urinary infection leading to high fever for a few days. This was brought under control with antibiotics, which were administered off and on for eight months to control the infection. We were advised to manually express her two or three times a day to prevent stasis of urine in the bladder. Quite by accident, we came to know that coconut water was an excellent diuretic, and thereafter we regularly gave her coconut water. Vigorous physiotherapy, such as the cycling movement and bending the legs up and down from the hips, also helped her to empty her bladder more fully, and we also gave her a lot of water to drink. All these helped in reducing stasis of urine.

Amba thereafter maintained steady progress, and crossed the various milestones easily. She was approximately nine months behind a normal child on some of the milestones, such as sitting up and crawling. Initially she used to propel herself on her stomach, but around the age of two she began to crawl on her knees. Originally she was taken to a hospital for physiotherapy by a trained physiotherapist every day, but when this became difficult, physiotherapy was continued at home, mainly by the mother and partly by a servant woman. The servant woman massaged Amba's body with warm oil before her bath – the traditional bathing routine for a baby in Indian homes.

The urinary infection keeps recurring every two or three months, but so far we have been able to control it without the use of antibiotics. On the advice of the orthopaedic surgeon, we fitted her with long leg callipers with a broad pelvic band when she was two years three months old. This enabled her to take a few steps with the aid of parallel bars. Today she can traverse the parallel bars up and down a number of times with ease.

So far there has been no evidence of any damage to the brain in spite of the hydrocephalus. Amba is an alert and cheerful child and eager to learn. She is good-natured and makes friends easily. Her vocabulary is increasing day by day. The orthopaedic surgeon told us nearly two years ago that if we could combat the urinary problem he saw no reason why by the age of twelve or thirteen Amba should not be able to walk independently with only a knee-length brace. With her spirit, and the way she cooperates with the therapists, she may well make it earlier.

The available literature and case histories on spina bifida children are almost entirely based on the experience of United Kingdom doctors, for as far as we know no record of the progress of spina bifida children in India has been kept. We therefore naturally had to rely on what the doctors told us or what we read in books written by British doctors. Indian doctors also, having mostly been trained in Britain, reflected the British view. From this standpoint, therefore, the progress made by Amba is remarkable.

If Amba's case is typical, then spina bifida children in India can fare better than their UK counterparts. The reasons, we believe, are as follows:

1. Since there is no National Health scheme and no specialist hospitals for spina bifida children in India, such children are brought up at home. The love and care that a baby gets at home from the parents, brothers and sisters, and often one or two other relatives, is something no hospital can match, however good it may be; the care bestowed by even the most devoted staff of a hospital is bound to be impersonal.

2. Our climate enables us to leave a baby without a napkin if need be for a few hours. This could be important in avoiding urinary infection.

3. Our climate also enables us to change the napkins as frequently as necessary, since washing and drying them is no problem.

4. The availability of domestic help enables the parents to give more time and attention to a spina bifida baby than is possible in the west. Amba's mother could spend three to four hours a day exclusively on the regimen of physiotherapy, massage and yoga for Amba.

5. With the baby being at home, we could adopt many unconventional and folklore cures. We had been told about coconut water by a chance acquaintance. A servant woman told us that the water in which rice is cleaned is good for development of the muscles, and we heat this rice water and pour it over Amba's legs at bath-time.

6. The yoga teacher, Yogacharya Janikiraman, who was

experimenting with the therapeutic aspects of yoga, and who had cured a number of people of chronic ailments such as hypertension, migraine, etc., took up Amba's case as a challenge, although he had not previously handled any spina bifida cases. We are confident that his advice and treatment have had a beneficial effect.

The Yoga Therapy prescribed by Janikiraman

Janikiraman asked Mrs Prabhala to bring her daughter to his house so that I could study the case and the effect of his treatment. Amba was 6½ years old, very sweet, small and pretty. Mrs Prabhala was dressed in a smart sari, was very friendly and was willing to pass on to us all the details about her daughter.

Janikiraman explained how rare spina bifida is in India, as it is generally found in colder countries such as the UK and Europe. The mother showed me where Amba's spine had been operated on to close the spine at the lumbar-sacral region. The scar extended from one side of the lower back to the other and went up the spine to the waist.

Janikiraman said, 'I did not know about such a case before this child was brought to me. Originally I received mother and child with love, the right method of conquering disease. Then I transferred this from the heart to the mind, through divine guidance. I had noticed that the child had a slightly delayed reaction, and her head was slightly larger than the normal. I was able to show the mother how she could control the child's nervous energy by silent communication, and by placing her hands gently on the child's head and reciting the sound 'OM'.

The mother said, 'Whenever Amba cried or was in pain, I noticed that the top of the head was very tense. Janikiraman had told me never to put my palms on the top of the head and I found I could comfort her by placing my palms on the sides of her head while softly humming the 'OM' vibration. In two or three minutes this always had a relaxing effect on the child, which helped me too.

'I had to measure the diameter of Amba's head and I noticed that it grew a little after the shunt was inserted, but it stopped growing when we started with the sound "OM". Another exercise Mr Janikiraman gave me was to have Amba stick her tongue out and say "Ha", which had a good effect on the functioning of the brain.'

Janikiraman had read up on spina bifida and learned about the operation that was performed. My explanation is taken from Black's Medical Dictionary and Gray's Anatomy: 'Spina Bifida – a condition in which the development of the spinal cord and its covering is incomplete. All degrees of defect occur, and shortly after birth it may be necessary to perform an operation to cover the incomplete part. Hydrocephalus is sometimes present in cases of spina bifida, and operations for both conditions may be required. Hydrocephalus is a condition in which there is an abnormal accumulation of cerebrospinal fluid within the skull. There are several different causes, and if it is not present at birth the hydrocephalus develops later. An operation is then performed to put a tube with a one-way valve into the brain to drain the excess fluid into the large veins of the neck or abdomen. When successful, this prevents the enlargement of the head, and may prevent further deterioration of the intelligence.'

Janakiraman said, 'Amba's parents told me that when she was born she had no reflex action in the lower legs. When she came to me there was no power flowing from the coccyx area which had been operated on, and it felt icy cold. This is actually the area which stores the shakti energy which is the primordial force behind all movement that is generated from the base of the spine. In the early days it was established that the child had very slight

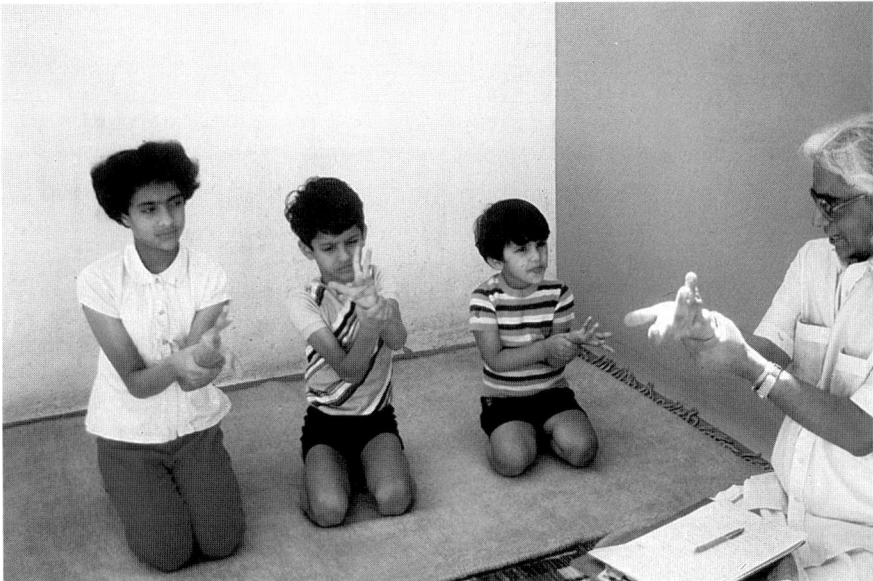

Janikiraman instructs his grandchildren to loosen the finger joints.

movement in her thighs and there was approximately 10–15 per cent movement in her legs.

I instructed the mother to have her lie face down on the floor and put her feet against the wall. Pressing her feet against the wall began to strengthen them, for this puts pressure on the lower back area and the shakti energy starts to flow.'

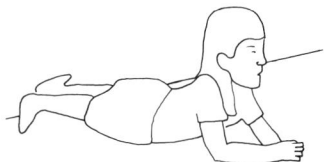

The next stage was to encourage the child to straighten her legs supported against the wall. We videoed Amba doing these leg movements. It was not easy for her, although Janikiraman said that she had now reached about 20–25 per cent movement in her legs.

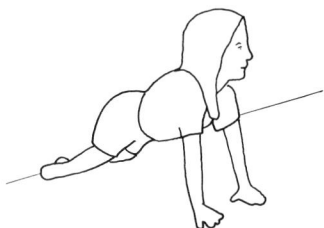

She tried to do the movement slowly, but there were some muscular spasmodic muscular jerks in her legs and she had no control whatsoever of her feet. Her feet kept flopping out sideways and Jana-kiraman kept telling her to keep her legs straight with her feet pressed against the wall.

This exercise built up the muscle tone, as well as awakening shakti. Eventually she managed to hold this position for about 30 seconds. These two movements were preparing her for Bhujunga-sana – the Cobra posture.

Janakiraman next told her to do the 'posture of the snake' for us. First she was to hold her arms straight out in front of her, then bring her hands back level with her shoulders, and then raise the elbows keeping them close to her body. After that she had to raise the upper part of her body, keeping her abdomen on the floor and bending at the waist. This concentrated pressure on the lower back and coccyx, and pushed the shakti energy down the legs.

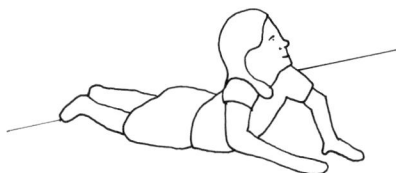

The mother said to me, 'Her legs have improved and there is sensation in the lower legs now, the same as she has always had in the upper thighs, but she still cannot move her toes at all'.

The next stage was to have Amba come up on to her hands and knees (four-footed posture) and rock forwards and backwards

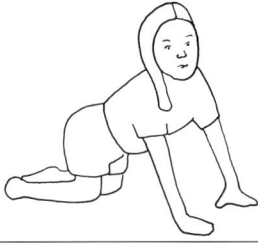

several times as a preparation for the Tiger Stretch, which involves articulating the vertebrae.

Janikiraman said, 'This is one of the most important and frequently used asanas in yoga therapy. This is because the spine takes on its natural curve, the shape it was meant to be. The reason why many spines are strained and weak is because the organs are under too much pressure. In the four-footed posture the abdominal organs are protected, and the heart is relieved of pressure so that it can function more effectively. When the static posture is held for a time, carbon dioxide is thrown off and this helps to relieve constriction in the chest area, which in turn helps to relieve asthma, heart problems, spinal complaints, abdominal and reproductive disorders.'

The next step was introduced because the mother found that sometimes Amba could not concentrate. Janakiraman showed them what he called the 'Head Pose' but what was in fact the Cat and Dog Stretch.

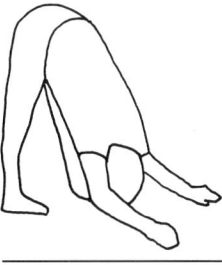

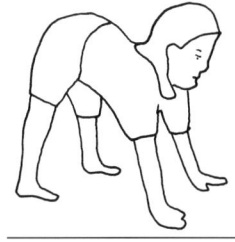

At the mention of the 'Head Pose' Amba moved from her four-footed posture and was able to straighten her legs a little. Although the right knee gave way several times, she diligently stayed in that position for a good two minutes. This was one of the newer exercises she had learnt.

The Cat and Dog inverted stretch posture invigorates the brain, promotes circulation throughout the extremities of the body and strengthens all the limbs.

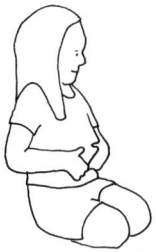

Following these movements, Janikiraman encouraged Amba to recite the 'AUM' sound. She placed her hands on her diaphragm and followed him in intoning long 'AUM' sound vibrations. When the sound 'AUM' reaches a certain resonance, its vibrations have the power to restore bodily harmony. It can resonate throughout the nervous system and affect first the area below the waist, and then the area above the waist up to the top of the head. In this way it can help to throw off negative forces that are active in the system. Just as the vibration of a car will throw off objects placed on the front window ledge, so will sound vibrations act on a damaged or diseased part of the body and perhaps disperse the cause. The sound 'AUM' has a rejuvenating effect on the whole person.

Mrs Prabhala remarked that what was still needed was something for Amba's incontinent bladder. Janikiraman rejoined that the bowel incontinence had been improved and it was only the lesser matter of the bladder which still needed treatment. He reminded her, 'Yoga therapy is a slow process and we must not be impatient. To build up the nervous system takes quite a time.' He recalled that originally there was no hope for the child. Then there were two risks involved: one was losing the power of movement through the closure of the spine, the other, the risk of an over-production of the cerebro-spinal fluid with resultant damage to the brain. He pointed out that the operation Amba had had did not damage her faculties but on the contrary enhanced them. She proved this by speaking two languages at the age of six and gaining more movement in her legs and control of her bowels. He urged the mother to focus her attention on Amba's remarkable improvement through yogic therapy, despite the prediction of the doctors that she would be mentally disabled (which she certainly is not). In this way he encouraged Mrs Prabhala to keep hopeful and positive, so that she would continue diligently with the yoga exercises so as to build up Amba's sacral area.

He also introduced mother and child to the sound 'Ha', done without sticking the tongue out (which was done in the early stage) to stimulate the brain centre. He made the sound forcefully, and told them, 'If you like, you can place your hands on your kidneys to feel the vibration of the sound striking that area. If practised several times a day, this sound will rejuvenate the kidneys and bladder.'

Janikiraman said that the family visits, which took place only once a month because they live so far away, were not frequent enough and that Amba would naturally improve more rapidly if she could see him daily. However, even with monthly visits he thought that Amba's bladder problem would improve in 2–4 years. Thus, by the age of ten, she should be cured of incontinence provided she continued to do her yoga regularly. By the age of thirteen or fourteen (which is the next stage of child growth) she might even attain the potential of being able to bear a child herself in due time.

Janakiraman pointed out that in India there is substantial genetic control in marriages because of the caste system. Some castes, the Brahmins for instance, know their ancestors' lineage going back for thousands of years. Within the caste they have family groups which avoid intermarrying, but if members should intermarry, this could cause genetic problems in the children. Janakiraman thought that this general rule might help to account for the rarity of spina bifida within the caste system. On the other hand, the 'Untouchables' (the poor who have to live in shacks or tents), who have no caste system, have a large number of children born with congenital defects. Of course malnutrition also contributes to this situation.

Mrs Prabhala admitted that she was from the same family group as her husband, with whom she had a blood relationship through her ancestors. She agreed that this could explain the unfortunate and unusual circumstance of her child's condition.

During our intensive training with Janikiraman, he also introduced us to the basic idea of the eight major sets of joints – the ankles, knees, hips, waist, wrist, elbows, shoulders and neck. This concept has since been the result of the twenty-two Looseners in

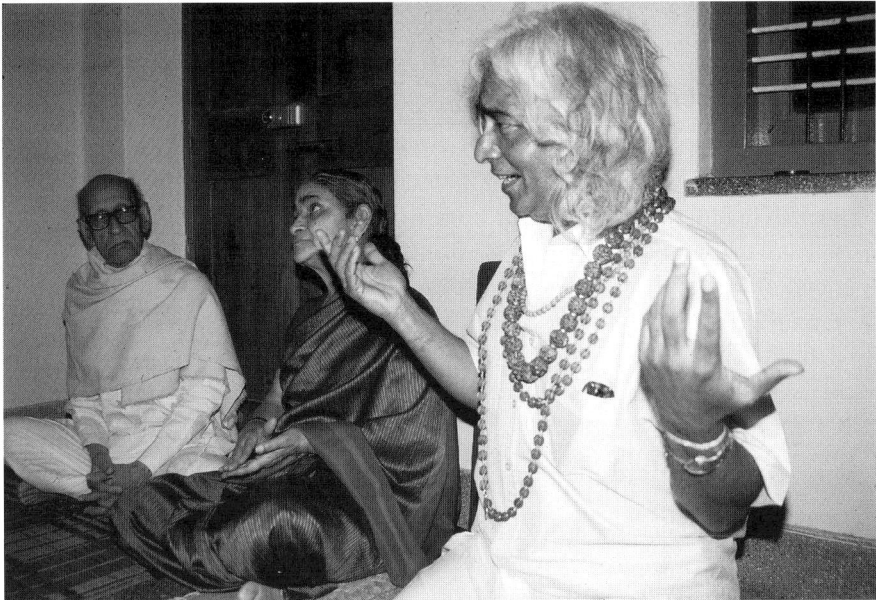

Janikiraman conducts Bhajana – devotional songs – at Atma Jyothi.

the YOU & ME system which are used for assessment as well as for loosening-up the joints. Janikirman demonstrated various movements for the eight joint areas for us to film. He was accompanied by his three grandchildren, aged 3, 7 and 11, and this took place on the roof top of his ashram.

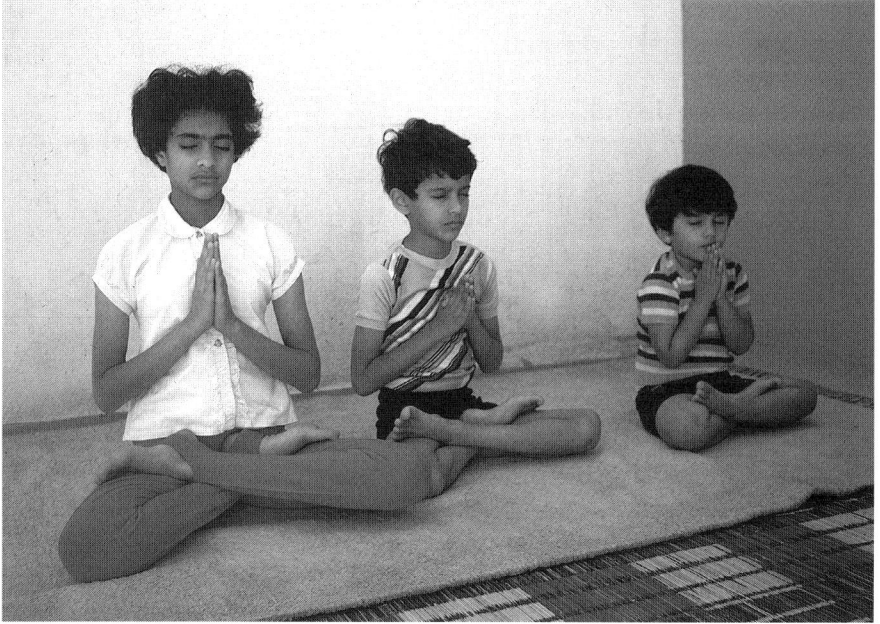

The children give thanks (Namaste).

I am deeply grateful for the generosity of the Winston Churchill Memorial Trust which gave me a unique opportunity to gain new knowledge and insights into a subject of such great value to disadvantaged members of society. I trust that what I learned directly from masters of yoga and others, in the great country whose ancient civilisation produced this wonderful philosophy and practical guide to wholesome living, may prove of continuing benefit not only to myself in my own work with disabled people, but also to teachers of yoga and others dedicated to helping the disabled fulfil their potential.

Part Three

After India

CHAPTER TWENTY

Life after my Indian Adventure

From my Fellowship I gained the confidence to widen my horizons and gain wide experience, not only in my own country, but internationally. I enjoy the two-way learning process of my work – there is always something new and exciting for each side to learn from the other. This is precisely how I have developed the YOU & ME system, by compiling and collating all the knowledge gained from everybody I have worked with – mainly good experiences, but occasionally painful learning experiences as well! Yoga embraces the whole subject of life and how to live it for the fulfilment of oneself and others. Yoga is very well suited to people with special needs because it enables everyone to help themselves and those with special needs usually have a strong desire for improvement. They are grateful for your teaching guidance or advice and compassionate friendship, and it is rewarding to teach such appreciative students.

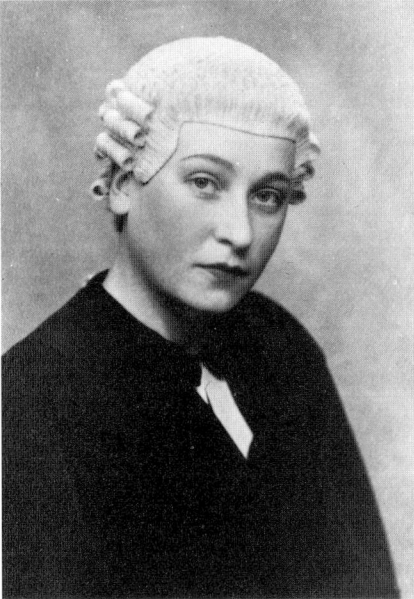

Beatrice Hope Alexander.

I am deeply grateful to the late Beatrice Hope Alexander, from the metaphysical group, who on my return from India showed a great interest in my Churchill Fellowship. I visited her home and spent hours with her going over experiences of my Indian adventure – investigating yoga for disabled people. She had an enquiring mind that delved deeply into facts and reason. This helped me sharpen-up my brain through thinking beyond just one's memory. She was my personal advisor for fourteen years, and was always there for me, eager to listen and advise.

Having been one of the few English female barristers in the early 1930s, Beatrice possessed an excellent command of the English language. We would sit side-by-side for anything up to four hours at a time going over my written work, discussing my ideas about yoga for people with learning difficulties. She had the art of keeping detail simple and was a poetical genious with insight, wisdom, style, charm and dedicated compassion for humanity as a whole. She was always so patient with me, an absolute angel in fact. Like a beacon of light she showed me how to progress intellectually beyond what I would have thought possible.

Following my return from three months in India, my special needs classes at Southwark had been changed which eventually led to the termination of my work. I was given three months' notice and my work conditions changed drastically. I was told it was due to the future closure of the ILEA and consequent pressure for 'cutbacks' that everyone seemed to be up against. Later I discovered that the Head of PE had unsuccessfully applied for a Churchill Fellowship that same year in Sports for the Disabled. I was unduly subjected to poor working conditions and had to carry equipment and drive a large van to ferry students to and from their yoga sessions, without assistance. Due to the strain on my neck, at the end of the session I temporarily lost the use of my right arm. After twelve years of building my strength through yoga practice this was quite a set-back for me and unfortunately has been my weakness ever since. My osteopath told me I should never again lift anything heavier than two bags of sugar and that I should give up teaching yoga or risk permanent paralysis. Consequently the following years have been a struggle, not only had I lost my core yoga group but also was up against bleak financial prospects in my career.

Since this time, I have not worked with disabled students in the same way as the neurological weakness in my arms would be under threat through possibly having to lift a disabled student. So there I was, very frustrated, with all the knowledge and experience from my Churchill Fellowship but without my core group of students with whom to work.

However, I was able to carry on working in integrated setups at the Hollies Home with carers and residents, and Sherard Road Centre with teachers and clients. I also worked with staff training at Grove Park Hospital, with RHMH student nurses and members of the OT department. We had intermittent integrated sessions with some patients and met every Friday for twelve weeks. This

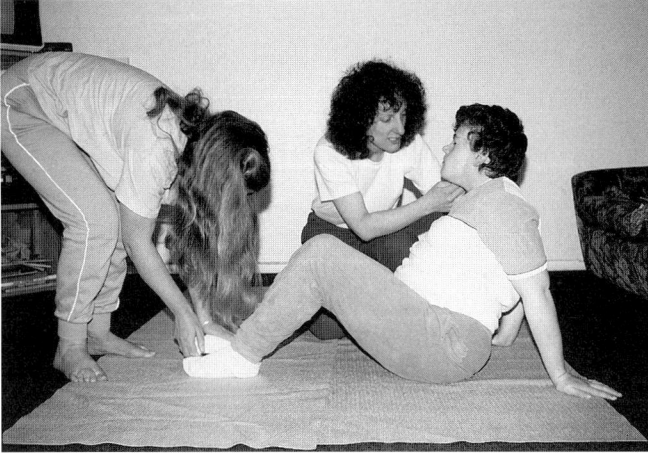

Two carers working with a resident at the Hollies.

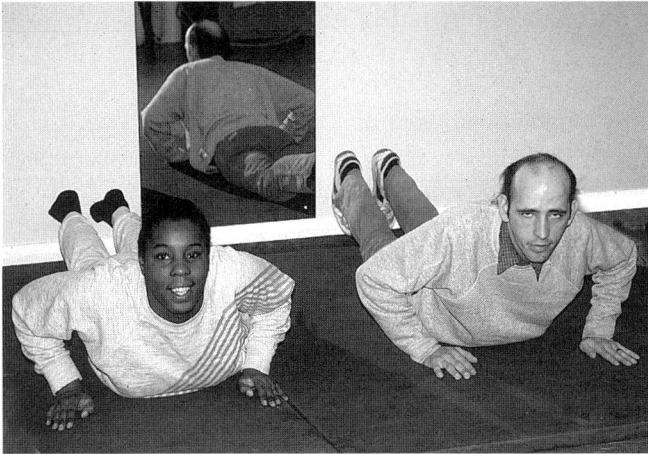

Students at Sherard Road Centre, with feet against the wall, practising the Cobra.

was valuable time to test out some of my new knowledge with some familiar staff as well as some new members.

The outcome was that staff enjoyed the practices, particularly the relaxation, but they were not interested in spending time learning the Sanskrit names of the techniques. Neither were they interested in learning about the origin of the techniques. This was because they were mainly concerned with learning techniques and methods to use with their patients. Thus, the use of the Sanskrit names of the yoga techniques has been changed, and over the years, appropriate names have been given to each of the YOU & ME techniques – names to which Westerners can relate. The YOU & ME Yoga system was consequently devised to pass on knowledge gained so that staff can practice yoga with special needs students.

According to MENCAP Information Services (2000), the number

of people in the UK with some degree of learning disability is estimated at 1.2 million – approximately 2 per cent of the total population. Therapists, staff and carers can learn from the YOU & ME programme what yoga techniques can be incorporated in their training as a valuable adjunct to existing provision.

Teaching in France

On two occasions my work took me to France. Mr Mahesh (Director, Centre De Relations Culturelles Franco-Indien, Paris), had contacted me through my article 'Yoga for Mentally Handicapped – Marvellous Human Beings' 1984, published in the newsletters from the Indian conferences I had attended the previous year. Mr Mahesh invited me to his Yoga Conference holiday weekends to introduce yoga for people with learning difficulties to his groups – mainly visiting yoga teachers from various parts of France. I informed Mr Mahesh that I would need someone to carry my bags and he allowed Chris to join me on two trips of luxury to St Baume in the south and Bitche in the north. At the magnificent monastery of St Baume there is a cave with a shrine where local tradition has it that Mary Magdalene stayed some years after the Crucifixion. At St Baume there were over three hundred yoga enthusiasts. Marcel, my interpreter repeated every couple of sentences in French. It was strange having my discourse punctuated in this way. The practical sessions were even more unusual as my instructions were interpreted to the groups by Marcel through a loudspeaker! Surprisingly this worked quite well. The outside session was really stunning. I asked the hundreds attending to form into groups of three, and allotted each one with the extraordinary experience of not being able to see, or hear, or speak. Once everyone had chosen their condition, they took it in turns to teach each other my instructions interpreted by Marcel. As you can imagine, most were hesitant at attempting a seemingly inconceivable role. However, soon everyone began to really get involved with their different roles and states of being, and experienced the difficulties encountered from such disabling conditions. When delivering the instructions, they were confronted with the challenge of finding ways of making themselves understood by others with some of their faculties missing. In this instance, communication was not a problem because of the care and concern expressed for one another. This was very moving.

Mr Mahesh invited yoga masters from all over to his conferences:

At St Baume, Mr Pandit from Sri Aurobindo Centre, Pondicherry was the main guest speaker. We had previously met Mr Pandit at the YOCOCEN conference. He spoke about Aurobindo's teachings that were carried out by 'The Mother' – Mirra Alfassa.

Sri Aurobindo, 1872–1950, was a great yoga philosopher and sage. He was world-famous for his enlightened view of yoga, and said of it, 'Yoga is not a thing of ideas, but of inner spiritual experience.' His law of life was for everybody to grow in his own way, 'to prosper or to perish'. He would never question that right. He said that true yoga does not require renunciation but enriches life with divine perfection, through an inner awareness, an overwhelming aspiration to overcome the temptation of evil forces and emerge fresh, unspoilt, untouched.

'The Mother' was a French lady named Mirra Alfassa who went to Pondicherry to meet Sri Aurobindo in 1914, when she was 34, and remained in his ashram until she died at the age of 95.

Chris and I stayed at the Aurobindo Centre in Delhi at the beginning of my Fellowship in December 1984. We were very impressed by their new age educational systems in the midst of a spiritual sanctuary. A full report about the Aurobindo Centre, and 'The Mothers' educational work is available on request.

During our visit to Bitche, Dr M V Bhole, M.D., whom we had met at Kaivalyadhama, was the main guest speaker. It was a wonderful opportunity to spend a few days getting to know Dr Bhole, who has kept in touch and contributed to the YOU & ME teachings. He has such a lot of experience and knowledge in explaining the workings and effects of yoga in scientific medical terms. During the practical sessions, Dr Bhole showed us how to use the breath and kriya (cleansing) techniques to revitalise the brain and to heal the body.

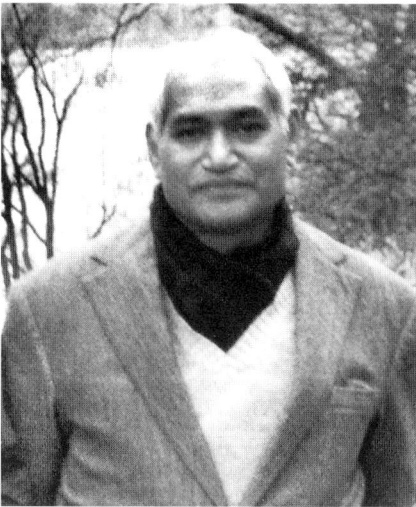

Dr Bhole regularly visits the West to share his scientific knowledge, wisdom and practical application of yoga. I can strongly recommend yoga enthusiasts to attend his sessions whenever possible. Dr Bhole has given me permission to reprint

Dr Bhole.

a chapter he wrote on 'YOGA', which was taken from the text book, 'Understanding Medical Physiology'. The editor of this work, Professor R.L. Bijlani, Head of Physiology, All India Institute of Medical Sciences, New Delhi, also gave me permission. There are three sections covering: Getting Introduced to Yoga; Physiological Understanding of Yogic Techniques; and Physiological Studies in Relation to Yoga and Meditation. This material was written for Medical Students, but would be suitable for serious academic yoga enthusiasts and further details are given at the end of this book.

A bit of a laugh

Sometime ago I was interviewed on Radio Lancashire about my work. In the interview I was asked to explain the difference between yoga and other forms of exercise and I mentioned the importance of breathing and relaxation. After some sarcasm about 'simple' breathing, my interviewer put me on the spot to prove how breathing can make you feel calm. I suggested he should experience the practice for himself and that the best position to do so would be lying on the floor. To everybody's surprise he got off his chair keeping his headphones on and laid down on the floor for what was quite a unique experience. I sat on the floor beside him, and spoke into the microphone gently about concentrating on the flow of his breath, the movement of his diaphragm and deepening the depth of his breathing, and instructed him to make the 'throat breath' sound. The sound crew and receptionists were all up at the window looking in amazement at us on the floor doing deep breathing. After a few rounds, I asked him to go back to normal breathing and remain still and quite for a moment. The whole studio became motionless. Then I quietly instructed him to wiggle his fingers and toes and open his eyes. He was surprised that he had managed to become so relaxed in just three minutes and acknowledged it must have been because of his control over his breathing!

My Personal Life

My health frequently reminds me not to push myself physically and I have found a lot of salvation through my yoga practice. I do most of my practice in bed in the mornings on waking by focusing on my breathing allowing the ebbing-and-flowing of the breath to come and go freely. I am sure that it is this powerful practice that has kept me from getting bogged down with the innumerable obstacles and challenges and helped me to keep my concentration on developing the YOU & ME yoga system over all these years.

I also do my meditation in the place where I feel most comfortable and relaxed – my bed. It is important to listen to your inner voice and not just follow automatically the rules laid down by other disciplines. Yoga is nowadays becoming a system of techniques based on the interchange of views and information among seekers on the spiritual path and shared with others. To discover what is right for you and make it your own sense of achievement and responsibility is ultimate self-development.

I prefer to meditate in the morning, sitting up in bed, and although I do practise some other times, morning is the time of day I find my mind is most active. This is more inviting than sitting on the floor on a cold morning. On one particular morning, I was just approaching a deep meditative state, when I felt one of my cats jump up on to the foot of my bed and start to make her way to me, pawing on the covers as she came. I knew this would have a disturbing effect on the quality of my concentration and meditation, so I built up a mental barrier of light around me. The cat came no further, but settled down a little away from me, purring contentedly, which I found as soothing and relaxing as she did!

One of the ancient traditions of yoga is to mentally put a circle of light around the solar plexus for protection. If someone is expressing antagonism towards you, you can clothe yourself completely in a cloak of light. This technique does not mean that you should blank the hostile person from your mind altogether, but just keep your channels of awareness open for your own needs. As a small illustration of the legitimate use of mental power, on one occasion my friend and her son with cerebral palsy – were joining me for a day's outing to the beach. We decided we'd meet on the 10a.m. bus. When I boarded the bus there was only the three-seater, opposite the entrance door, available. My friends were not joining the bus until two stops further on. At the next stop two young men boarded the bus separately. They both looked at the unoccupied seats, obviously considering whether to claim them. In each case I mentally directed them to the upper deck, and after a moments hesitation, they both went upstairs. Thus, I saved my friends the inconvenience of not being able to board the bus and we arrived early enough for the best days' sunshine. I was relieved not to cause any inconvenience and the day was really enjoyable.

Mental power can always be used in this way provided it is for a good, positive purpose and cannot harm anyone else. This remains in my memory as a small but forceful demonstration of the power of the mind to control and direct the subtle energy fields that surround us.

Although this may seem trivial and mundane, at the time I felt the power of my mind put me in control. It is comforting to know that sometimes you can achieve what you want when you need it. I've been told by my friends and teachers – Valerie and David Tarbuck, that the 'law of attraction' draws to us that which is like our thought. The more we focus our thoughts upon good the more we draw good things towards us.

In point of fact, I have used the mental barrier of light when bees or wasps try to approach me and it always keeps them a reasonable distance away from me, for there is enough room for them as well as me.

Observing animals in their movements is quite an inspiration. By instinct they have their own exercises to do for keeping supple and well. My tortoise was given to me when my lovely Nan died. We call her Lub and she's been in the family for 28 years. I have spent a lot of time meditating with Lub, being with her in her stillness and peaceful atmosphere. She shows me how she performs her YOU & ME Yoga by gently pumping her front legs back and forth which makes her breathe deeper as she coordinates moving her legs with puffing sounds.

I also have several cats who join in with the yoga by showing me how to really relax. When doing my postures in the garden, my cats are usually sitting close by and on occasions I am shown how to cat-stretch when they get up from their slumber. Yoga is not just the practice of techniques, it is a process of getting to know yourself and your relationship with life. Nature can help to show us how precious life is.

Yoga is a wonderful way of life. On early sunny mornings when the sun is shining gloriously warm, I do my yoga practice in the garden. This usually involves doing the Salute to the Sun, Postures, Neck Rolls, Alternate Nostril Breathing, Mudras, Full Lung Breathing, Relaxation and Meditation. During my meditation I often become aware of the birds singing and the expanse of space all round me, of which I feel so privileged to be an integral part. I enjoy having my peaceful garden where we grow our own vegetables and fruits. There is so much life-force which bursts forth from freshly picked food – the life giving substance of purity in perfection.

Yoga has been a major part of my life which started when I was twenty following a serious car accident and since then my life has evolved through different aspects of yoga as follows:

1. Improving my health through regular practise of Hatha (physical posture) Yoga to increase flexibility and stamina.

2. Recognising healing taking place in my body through conscious relaxation techniques by becoming still, aware and revitalised. (Yoga Nidra.)

3. Supporting my mental and emotional needs through Pranayama (breath control) and increasing my vitality and ability to focus and to be calm with a sense of harmony within.

4. Overcoming amnesia through constant remembering and mindfulness techniques improving my ability to concentrate introspectively. (Pratyahara – withdrawing the five physical senses, and Dharana – concentration.)

5. Building my confidence through teaching Yoga. (Karma yoga – cause and effect.)

6. Applying selflessness and humanity through sharing my benefits of practice with other disabled people and their carers. (Bhakti – yoga of love).

7. Developing awareness of my thinking through 'Science of Mind'. (Raja yoga is the yoga of the mind.)

8. Broadening my education and social skills through my Travelling Churchill Fellowship in India. (Meeting the great Yoga Masters.)

9. Intellectual development through writing about my investigations in India, inspired by the enthusiasm and guidance of Beatrice Hope Alexander (personal advisor).

10. Acquiring analytical skills through synthesising my yoga knowledge and experience into the comprehensive YOU & ME Yoga programmes for students, trainers and tutor trainers. This motivated me to endure my mission, even though it unexpectedly took several years to accomplish. (Jnana – yoga of knowledge; Dhyana – contemplation.)

11. Attunement with my environment and experience being one with the universe through meditation. (Laya – yoga of merging of the Mind.)

12. Developing a training network in order to develop professional relationships among those who practise YOU & ME Yoga. (Bhavna – yoga of thinking, feeling and reasoning to reach the final aim).

I am sure there will be those who will shine through to train the future Tutors of Trainers, which will mean the YOU & ME system shall reign beyond my mission this lifetime! Then I should like to think I shall reach a state of contentment. (Samadhi – Bliss ecstasy).

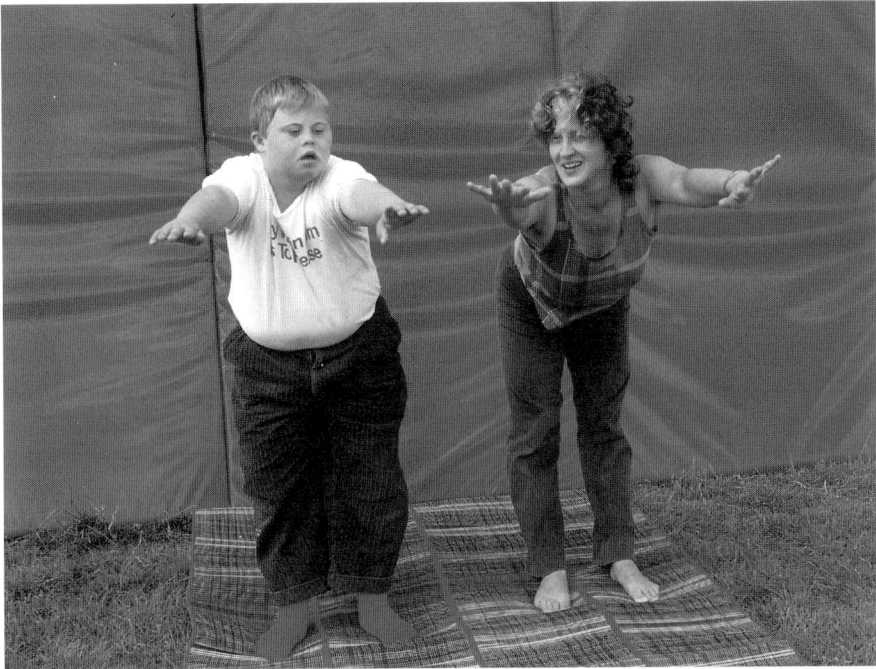

Reaching out together.

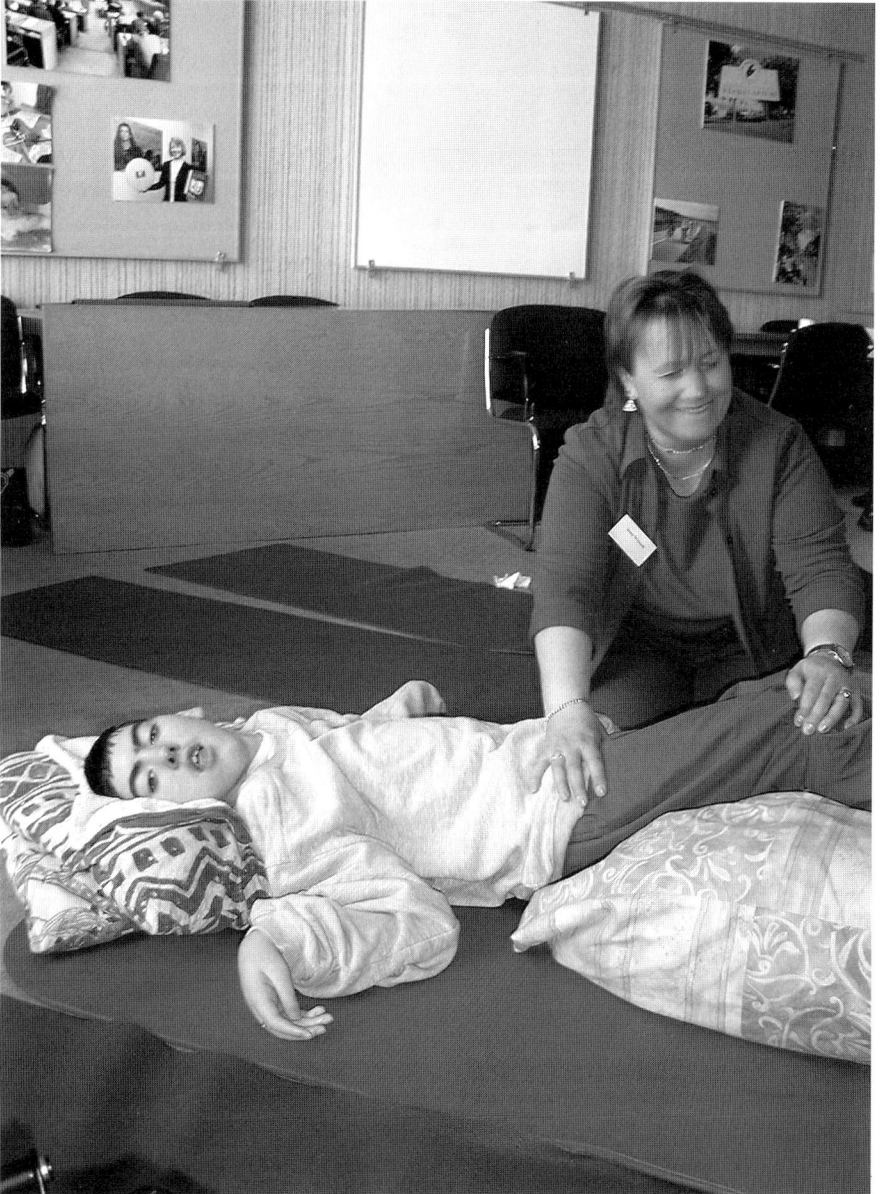

Jenny with her son Craig at a YOU & ME training course
held by PAMIS (Profound and Multiple Impairment Service).

Part Four

Developing the System

CHAPTER TWENTY-ONE

Development of the YOU & ME Yoga System

T hrough teaching yoga in the UK to various personnel and parents of persons with learning difficulties since 1978, the YOU & ME system has evolved. Originally I called the yoga system of sound, colour and movement 'YOU & ME', in preference to the more detailed and more cumbersome description of 'yoga integration training for trainers of persons with learning difficulties', because this simple phrase is one which students with learning difficulties can readily relate to. I have also used it as an acronym for the words 'Yoga Open Unfolding & Meaningful Experience', which genuinely describe the inner development that can take place through the practice of the YOU & ME techniques. The words 'YOU & ME' also fit in with the concept of yoga as meaning 'union'.

In 1988, at the time of inception, I started teaching YOU & ME to staff in Special Schools, Daycentres, Homes and Hospitals, on 'taster days', two-day, and three-day training courses as part of in-service training for staff at their workplace and various residential training centres throughout the country. During those courses, and other courses held in residential training centres, the YOU & ME system was developed to meet the individual needs of persons with learning difficulties and support the learning of people with a range of developmental needs and abilities.

In different parts of the United Kingdom and the Republic of Ireland, YOU & ME has been taught, by teachers whom I have trained, to thousands of students with special educational needs ranging from profound and multiply disabled students to students with mild learning disabilities. These include students with Down's Syndrome, autism, cerebral palsy, epilepsy, spasticity, paralysis, visual, aural and speech impairment, and psychiatric and/or behavioural problems.

Working with different people and groups, I have learned from their questions what next to work on and include in the system, i.e. what postures to use, when to do the practices, and how to practise. The YOU & ME system has been developed through listening, discussing, corresponding, analysing, sharing ideas, and offering learning opportunities to one and all. I have always been very ready to respond to suggestions for improving the system, which usually means simplifying the knowledge and the techniques.

The Postures have been given animal and other names for ease of identification. When practising with students instead of saying 'Breathe out' (as like the Indian system) we say 'ah' for

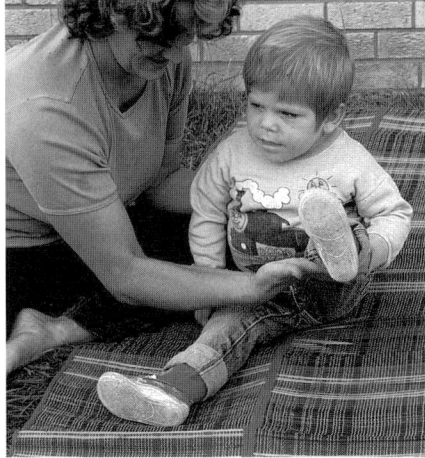

Young student assisted in doing the Rod.

the outbreath, which enables them to perform in unison, and assists them to breath correctly in coordination with their body movements. Uttering the names of the Postures, together with animal sounds is also used to assist breath and body coordination, where appropriate. Correct breathing helps to clear toxins from the body, reduces anxiety, and imparts a new sense of control which increases students' confidence and general wellbeing.

From research and experience I found that no one posture

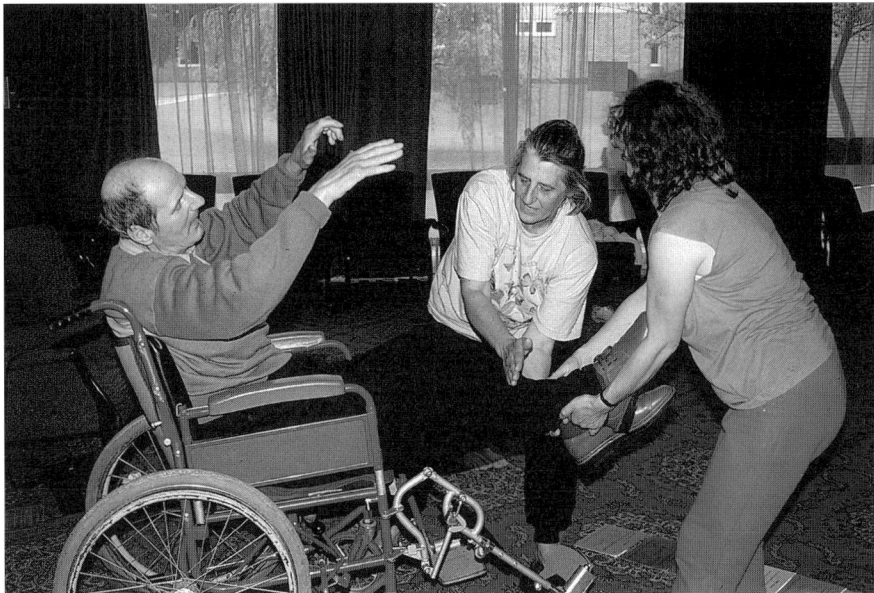

A student in a wheelchair assisted in doing the Crocodile's Mouth.

(asana) has a specific therapeutic effect for it is necessary to tone up all the bodily functions by using a series of movements for each of the main body areas. I devised the YOU & ME Whole-Body-Movement system comprising of carefully selected and arranged techniques which do not require much balance or physical effort, so as to be within the capacity of students with learning disabilities.

Whole-Body-Movement is designed to exercise and strengthen the different parts of the body by means of carefully chosen and arranged sequences of movement. In 1986, with the help of Tom Williams, Snr. Educational Psychologist, we devised the phrase 'Whole-Body-Movement' as a suitable name for a movement system for the whole body.

The sequencing of Postures in the system is based on the principle of Vinyasa which is based on Desikachar's organised structured approach, implemented in the Indian Special Needs curriculum, 1985. It involves a sequence of Postures from warming-up, through a main posture, and then winding down. As mentioned, based on the effective Indian system, we use sound to help the students breathe correctly and in unison. Relaxation is also an integral part of the system.

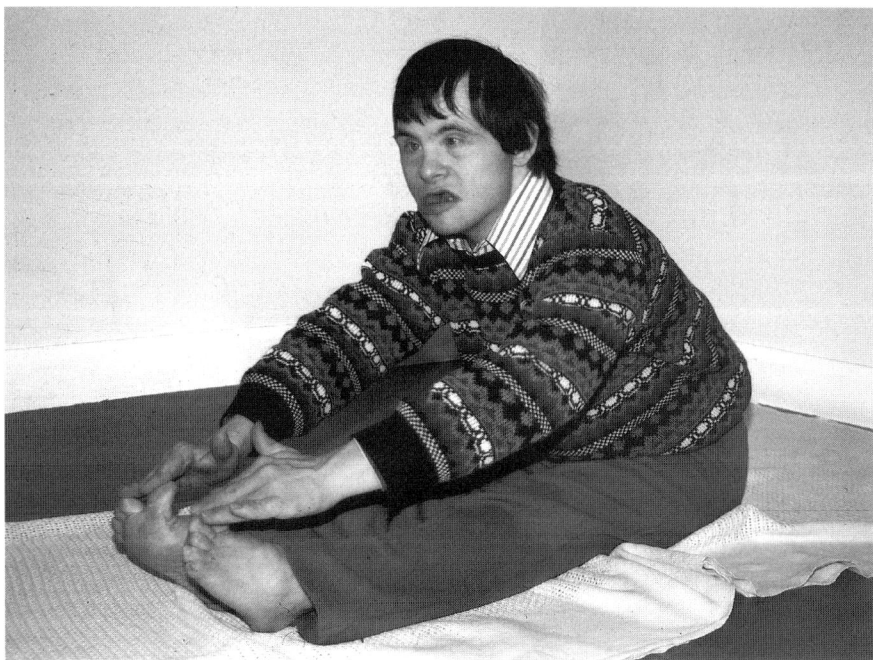

Eddie performing the Crocodile's Mouth.

Colour

According to James Hartley (1978), colour is the best medium through which people can be motivated to learn. Colour was introduced to me on a study-skills course I once attended where we were instructed to use coloured felt-tip pens to distinguish different sources of information, thus showing the effective use of colour for separating one meaning from another. The use of colour in the YOU & ME yoga system helps the students to understand that yoga is a meaningful experience for the whole of their being. The legs are coloured red, and the hips and lower back are orange. The waist and mid-back are yellow and the chest and upper back are green. The arms are coloured blue.

The indigo and violet colours represent the mindful aspect of movements. Indigo represents the movement of one side of the body being coordinated with the other. Colouring of one (left) arm as indigo represents the concept of awareness of each side in turn. Violet represents the characteristic of body awareness. The colouring of one (left) leg as violet represents the concept of awareness right down the full length of the body.

The seven colours of the spectrum, used in the YOU & ME teaching materials to identify the seven different coloured areas of the body, are useful to people with learning disabilities because even though they may not be able to communicate through language, they can more usually recognise colours. When teaching yoga to people with learning disabilities, the use of colour helps distinguish the different parts of their body. There is usually difficulty with distinguishing right and left sides. It is not unusual for students to get certain fixations and this can be expressed in isolated areas of their lives and bodies. Shifting attention from one part of the body to another makes it easier for students to become more receptive and alert, and to adapt to change within both the body and the mind. In this way life energy circulates, and consciousness is stimulated between mind and body. This is when yoga movement becomes more than a physical exercise, because there is a blending process of different aspects of a person's being, resulting in an unfolding meaningful experience.

When choosing the appropriate spectrum colour for each of the twenty Postures, the following points were considered for the performance of each Posture in the usual way:

- Which part of the body is mainly involved and has to be used when performing a particular Posture?
- Which part of the body is mainly affected by performance of that Posture?
- Can the Posture be performed even if the part of the body involved is not functioning properly?

When the colouring of the Postures was established, selection for a sequence of appropriate Postures was made much simpler and the outcome was the YOU & ME Colour-Code Instruction Pack for devising individualised programme plans of Whole-Body-Movement. In this system, a Main Posture is chosen to exert a particular coloured part of the body which needs to be developed. Each sequence is arranged around the Main Posture starting with Warming-Up movements selected to exercise the coloured parts of the body which are used for the performance of the Main Posture. The Main Posture is followed by Winding-Down movements, in the remaining spectrum colours, to complete the sequence.

Further Progress

There are twenty-two Looseners included in the system designed to loosen-up the eight major sets of joints before moving on to perform the Postures. Each Loosener has been colour-coded to correspond with the coloured area being worked on. This determines the degree of flexibility in a particular body area and indicates whether it would be appropriate to practice the related coloured Posture. With a thorough understanding of the YOU & ME colour-coding, it is possible to organise a sequence of movements for the whole body (which include both Looseners and Postures) that would be safe and suitable for any particular individuals' abilities.

There have been many course members including special needs teachers, carers and yoga teachers and other therapists, along with various disabled people, who have contributed to the development of this system. When showing course members the 20 Postures, it was decided not to use the classical yoga names of the Postures, but to substitute names to which students could relate. I asked the groups if they could consider what the Postures looked like, or what they brought to mind, and this produced the following:

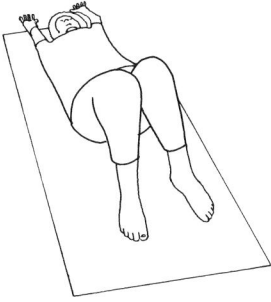

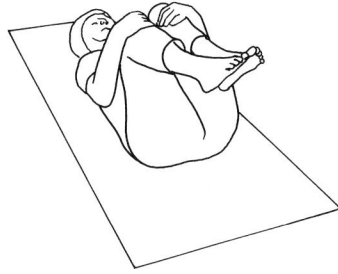

The Apanasana – a technique involving bringing the knees to the chest and what is referred to as the 'Gas Extractor'. A middle-aged member of a group suggested it reminded him of recently having his car wheel clamped, and so this Posture became the Clamp.

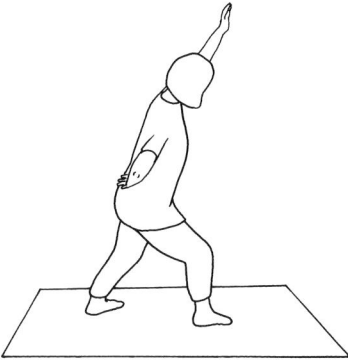

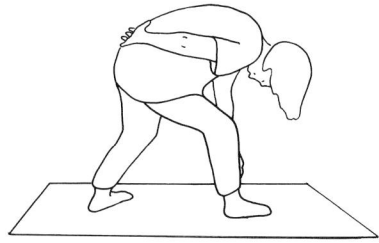

The Parsvottanasana – the widely used translation for this Posture is the Crane. This Posture reminded some staff of an elephant's trunk, when the arm was lowered, and they felt their students would enjoy making the sound of an elephant. And so the Crane is also known as the 'Elephant's Trunk'.

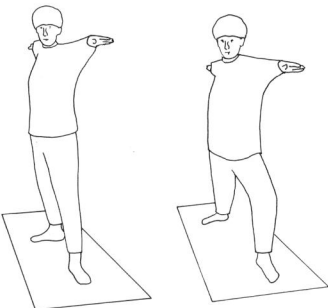

The Viradhadrasana – the Warrior – when performed a teacher used the sound 'Geronimo', when bending the knee into Posture; and we have since found that this sound instead of 'ah' can be suitably used with some students. Interestingly, Geronimo was a red Indian Warrior.

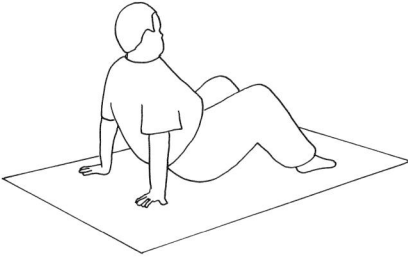

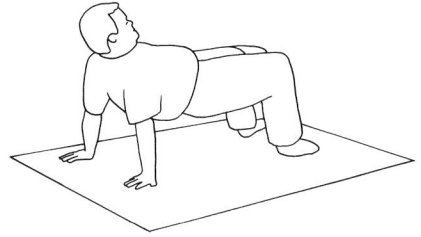

The Dandasana – the Table – was suggested by a physiotherapist from County Durham who realised that it can be used to help students to get up off the floor into a standing position, or into a wheelchair etc. The Table Posture makes use of the arms in an unusual way which in turn strengthens them.

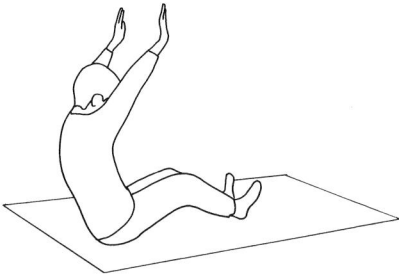

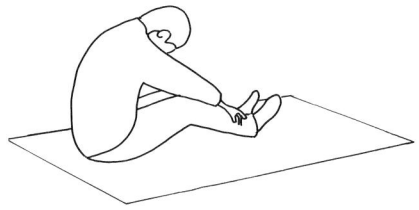

The Paschimottasana – the widely used translation for this is 'Sitting Forward Bend', but to make it more meaningful for our students, it was suggested by a course member that it should be called the 'Crocodile's Mouth', because it reminded them of the opening and shutting of the mouth of a crocodile. Because of this, some students like to say 'snap" rather than 'ah' as the arms are lowered.

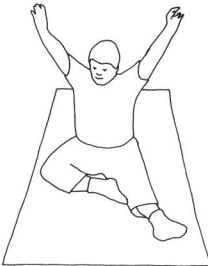

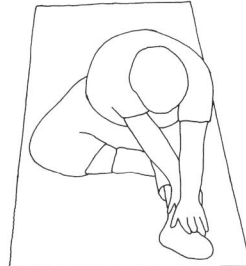

Janusirasana – the widely used translation is 'Head to Knee' – needed to be given a meaningful name. This proved to be quite difficult because it looks similar to the Crocodile's Mouth

Posture, yet one knee is bent out to the side, with the foot placed on the inside of the opposite thigh, which gives more ease in the hips. There is a Posture called the Butterfly in which both knees are bent out to the side with the soles of the feet touching; consequently the name 'Half Butterfly' is used. Additionally one arm is taken across the body to the opposite leg. When raising and lowering the arm it resembles the wing of a butterfly, and some students relate well to saying 'flutter, flutter, flutter', instead of saying 'ah' while breathing out and lowering the arm to the leg.

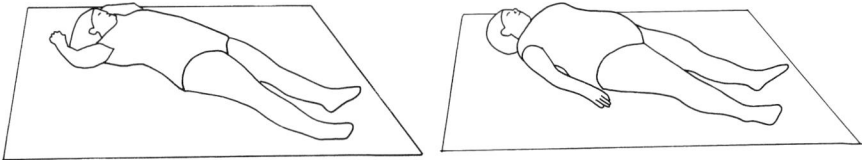

Savasana – the 'Corpse', a lying relaxation position – is a name a lot of people do not particularly like using, and another name that we found more suitable is 'Sleeping Beauty', because of the serenity on people's faces when they are in a state of deep relaxation.

The text of the instructions given on the Display Cards, used when teaching the Looseners and Postures, was settled by communicating with staff of students with varying ability and ages. I asked if they thought their students would be able to understand certain terms. The challenge of making the instructions simple enough for most students to follow, was considered by several of us over a long period. With this support, the instructions for the basic techniques given on the Display Cards have been established. Of course, language variables may always be used if more appropriate for particular students.

The YOU & ME system is non-competitive and allows each student to develop at their own pace, one to one, or in a group. Parents have given favourable reports on their children being easier to get on with when practising the system and they are amazed at the children's discipline in practising at home from their individual programme plans.

YOU & ME training involves techniques which are suitable and beneficial for staff and parents to practise with their charges. It is not necessary to have had any previous experience of yoga in order to train in the system. It is one of the satisfying by-products of teaching YOU & ME Yoga that practitioners find, as their work progresses, that they benefit along with their students. The system is also helpful for anyone who wishes to develop their potential still further by learning and practising techniques which enable mind and body to work in harmony.

The system has been specially adapted to the requirements and culture of the West. The training is unique in that it provides an additional dimension to the ordinary professional range of physical training and the everyday activities of people with learning disabilities.

I have found the system helps many types of conditions. For example, an elderly lady of 82 (who wished to be anonymous in my book), kindly allowed me to publish the beneficial and thera-peutic effects she gained from her daily YOU & ME Yoga practices with me, following a stroke she had which left her with slight hemiplegia on her left side. She regained her mobility and con-fidence to go out of the house and by the fifth month was determined to be fully independent again. She asked my husband, Chris, to accompany her in the car since she was unsure whether she was able to drive since the stroke. Her ability and skills to drive on the main road, her judgement of distance and coordination were restored within ten minutes. The lady was justifiably overjoyed at the sense of achievement, personal freedom and active social life she had retrieved since the stroke. She was convinced that the YOU & ME Yoga sessions had helped her make a speedy recovery. This incident made me realise how YOU & ME Yoga is suitable for other types of disabilities, no matter the age or ability, providing the person is prepared to practise with the will to get better.

YOU & ME Whole-Body-Movement Calendar

In 1989 I produced the YOU & ME Whole-Body-Movement Calendar. This teaching aid was aimed at encouraging the necessary motivation and discipline needed for practice of Whole-Body-Movement at home or in class. It illustrated a complete balanced yoga programme of the twenty Postures performed by persons with learning difficulties, right across the age range. These programmes were arranged in appropriate sequences of seven coloured Postures to benefit each of the seven coloured bodily areas.

The calendar provided a description of the Main Posture in the appropriate colour. Each illustration indicated the correct way to breathe into and out of each movement, along with the bodily area to be strengthened.

Each of the 52 weeks for the 1990 Calendar were arranged in a sequence of Whole-Body-Movement. The coloured Main Posture changed as the months went by, with the next spectrum colour up to end of seventh month of July and the remaining 21 weeks given a new spectrum coloured Main Posture each week up to the last week of December. A mathematical miracle!

YOU & ME Yoga Centre

For 1990 I was fortunate to be offered use of an unused barn which became the official YOU & ME Yoga Centre. After some minor decoration, it became a conducive environment in which to teach yoga. Several YOU & ME courses took place with small groups of people – mainly staff working in Special Needs including therapists, teachers and carers. A few parents brought their children for private consultation, which was thoroughly rewarding to see. It was my intention to involve parents and other family members with the practice, so that they could practise at home with their children at their convenience. A television crew, from Border Television's 'Lookaround' news programme, interviewed me and filmed a session with a class of local juniors from the local Burton Morewood School.

Ann Dixon, a mother from Bolton comments:

'I have made occasional visits to Maria with my 29-year-old daughter Louise, who has multiple disabilities. Louise practises nearly every day in her bedroom with either my husband or myself. We have been very pleased with Louise's increased flexibility and confidence. We hope to continue with the unique system of YOU & ME Yoga, which is specially designed for people like Louise.'

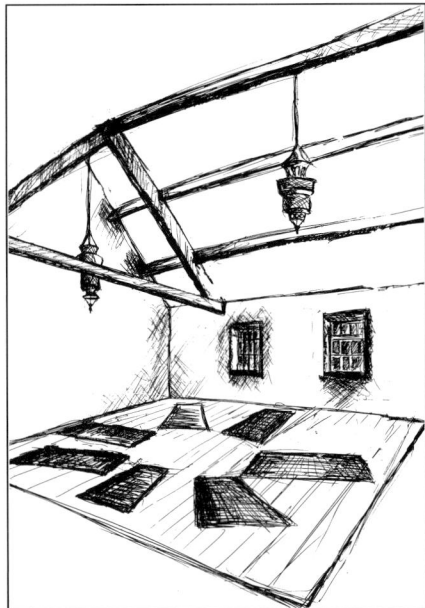

The YOU & ME Yoga Centre.
Drawing by Pauline Needham.

Louise Dixon adds:

'I follow my coloured Display Cards which I keep in my bedroom; they help me to be aware of the different parts of my body. I think the yoga is very good and it helps me a lot, I really enjoy the practice.'

Teaching Video

I decided to develop the YOU & ME teaching resources to reinforce learning of the system. With the help of a grant from Mencap City Foundation in 1992, I produced a teaching video showing people with learning difficulties of all ages and abilities demonstrating the system's techniques and the resultant benefits – increased mobility, improved dexterity, ability to relax and sit still, to concentrate, and to interact and cooperate with others.

Lancaster District Hospital Television (LDHTV) allowed me to use their filming equipment and editing studio to make this video. Five voluntary cameramen, including Chris, did 55 hours filming over a period of two years at nineteen UK and Eire centres – including special schools, residential homes, hospitals and adult training centres. I edited the film with some technical assistance from Bill Livesey, Studio Manager of LDHTV, and this resulted in a 140-minutes teaching video – quite a marathon! Isobel Hamid, a semi-professional speaker, generously did the voice-over for the video.

On the YOU & ME Whole-Body-Movement Teaching Video you can see John from Hensingham who could originally only balance by leaning against the wall. From regularly attending Elaine Harding's YOU & ME Yoga sessions one-hour each week for a few years he was able to stand with raised arms and balance without support. Sheila from the same group improved her coordination to eventually perform the indigo Half Butterfly Posture (a cross-lateral movement) by following verbal instructions even without imitating her teacher's demonstration.

The following extract was published in Yoga and Health magazine, October 1991.

Pauline Mifflin explains about her teaching experience of the YOU & ME Whole-Body-Movement at Mayfield School, Whitehaven.

As a practitioner and teacher of yoga for many years, as well as being a teacher in a school for pupils with severe learning difficulties, I was interested to find out about the YOU & ME yoga system. A colleague and I attended one of Maria's residential training courses which completely revolutionised my approach to teaching yoga to students with learning difficulties. It opened up a whole new approach which incorporated several areas of the National Curriculum. Also, we have been able to adapt it to the needs of the most profound and multiply-disabled students, because YOU & ME actively encourages the development of awareness of self, fine and gross motor skills, balance, hand/eye coordination, concentration and the ability to realise the difference between tension and relaxation.

Additionally, for those students with behavioural problems, we have noted that the practice of breath control and relaxation has had a noticeable effect on their ability to calm themselves down more quickly. This of course helps develop self-control, confidence and self-esteem.

So how did we approach the 'Whole-Body-Movement' at Mayfield School? We decided that the colour, sound and movement system lent itself to a cross-curricular project, covering National Curriculum attainment targets in English, Maths, Science, plus Geography, Arts and Crafts and Personal and Social Education.

Our first session was both practical and messy! We made a life-size cardboard cut-out of one of our students, then painted it to match the YOU & ME spectrum coloured chart. This chart has been used in every subsequent lesson to focus attention on the significance and relationship between the colours and body parts to be worked on.

During the second term, students learnt to recognise the postures on the Display Cards, to match the coloured cards to body parts, and to work on the relevant coloured postures. We kept to the same routine after choosing an appropriate sequence so that the students became familiar with a set format. And they love it! Especially the sounds we all make as we breathe out. The system allows them to participate in the learning process as we discuss together how best to adapt a posture to suit a particular individual. It has been very satisfying listening while students contribute to these sessions, making suggestions, correcting each other's postures, or complementing each other on their achievements.

It is noticeable how many other members of staff in school remarked upon the improvement, particularly in concentration and relaxation which they have observed in this group. I myself am convinced of its merit, and so are my students.

The students learned to associate the relevant colours with the various body parts. I was particularly pleased with the way they became familiar with the colour coding, recognising postures from the coloured cards and making good attempts to perform the postures from the illustrations. They gelled together as a group, and gradually felt confident enough to demonstrate the postures and even correct each other's mistakes, but also were quick to compliment each other for a posture well done, or suggest a different way of doing it if it proved too difficult. Another noticeable benefit of the system has been the calming affect the breathing and relaxation has had on the hyperactive students and those with behavioural problems.

Further case studies which may be of interest

One student, Jane, has athetoid cerebral palsy. She told the trainer who works with her on a one-to-one basis about the things she especially wanted to achieve – to be able to sit up straighter and hold her head up. Having a typical extensor thrust of chin, she suffered a good deal of neck-ache. She also hoped to gain more control of her arms for eating and drinking, and using her Makaton signing. Toileting was a problem. She found it uncomfortable to be handled by various staff assistants and wanted to be able to pull herself up out of her wheelchair and go to the toilet without help. After six months of regular YOU & ME practice, she was able to achieve all these objectives through her personal Whole-Body-Movement programme devised by herself and her trainer, Pat, who describes this practice in the YOU & ME Handbook, 'Learning Difficulties/Disabilities and Associated Conditions'.

Two contrasting reactions to the YOU & ME basic relaxation have been noted. One is a young man with Down's syndrome who speaks very little, and the other, a young woman who is hyperactive and nervous. He enjoys the other members' silence and by sitting quietly with them, contributes to the unity of the group. She on the other hand originally could not stay quiet for more then a few minutes, before she jumped up and rushed out of the class. Over many weeks we found that she responded to a male trainer, but not to female trainers, when asked to rejoin the class. To avoid her being too dependent on the male trainer, the female trainers made a point of teaching her for part of the time. After the fifth week she was able to stay for the full session and participate in the class. Rather surprisingly, the rest of the group have not been disturbed by her behaviour, but have been even more concentrated and relaxed – to counterbalance the disturbance, so to speak.

For seven years, from 1987, I introduced the YOU & ME yoga system to over two thousand carers, parents and therapists. The following are various comments about these courses:

Dr Roy McConkey, Border Region, Scotland, Brothers of Charity Service:

'Following the YOU & ME training, yoga features in our day-centre programme for clients with severe learning difficulties. We have seen improvements in their concentration, socialisation and relaxation, as they have mastered a range of yoga movements.'

Clive Ingram, Gateway Development Officer, Inner London:

'The YOU & ME system of Yoga has unfolded a new and exciting aspect of yoga for me. It is unique in that it simplifies many postures while still retaining their effectiveness, having a gentle yet profound effect on the whole body. It provides an excellent structure for using yoga with people who have learning difficulties, however severe.'

Lynn Bhania, Special Teacher, Radlett Lodge (Autistic School), Herts:

'The pupils enjoy it because they smile and laugh. They sustain concentration for longer periods than normal, and do not wander off or become disruptive. They watch each other and try to work together as well as making appropriate sounds when asked. They seem better able to coordinate their bodies when performing the movements, and feel secure in the structure imposed by the pictures, YOU & ME cards, and familiar routines. Obsessional and ritualistic behaviours are decreased during the session, and a general air of calmness and control seems to prevail.'

Sally Maloney, Coordinator, Stanchester Community School, Somerset:

'A most successful and beneficial course, and we are 100 per cent behind the aims of this system.'

As time went by, I became concerned that people were doing one, two or maybe three days' training with me, then going away and training others in what they were calling the YOU & ME yoga system. I did not know which techniques they were using or whether they were teaching them competently. This was rather alarming as if the techniques had not been mastered, a disabled person may have been injured, and the reputation and validity of my system compromised. Consequently, I devised the competence-based training programmes.

Vocational Qualifications

I wanted to ensure that people teaching the YOU & ME system meet national standards and that only those who genuinely meet the requirements be accredited with a certificate of competence for their teaching. To this end, competence-based programmes in the YOU & ME Whole-Body-Movement for Students, Trainers and Tutor Trainers have been approved by the Open College of the North West (OCNW).

It was decided with the OCNW that the best route would be to discover whether students with learning difficulties and/or disabilities could demonstrate competence in the YOU & ME techniques. In Autumn 1993 a competence-based programme was submitted with the following outcome:

Testimonial by Jakes Makin, Inter College Coordinator, November 1993 states:

> The Open College of the North West has recognised, approved and accredited the pre-vocational YOU & ME Whole-Body-Movement Training. We should like to advise the Department of Employment to accept this course aimed at people with learning difficulties/disabilities, for a number of reasons:
>
> - it improves awareness and concentration
> - it raises physical skill levels and confidence
> - it addresses the individual needs of students with a range of developmental needs and abilities.
>
> The above appear to us to be necessary prerequisites for such people to progress towards learning and training for independent living and employment. The course has genuine credentials as a pre-vocational provision.

YOU & ME Trust

In 1995 the YOU & ME Trust was formed to pilot programmes and provide opportunities for people with learning difficulties/disabilities to share and develop skills in YOU & ME practices. In accordance with the YOU & ME Trust Deed, the main object and activity was for the benefit of persons with learning difficulties and/or disabilities – in particular by the provision of YOU & ME Whole-Body-Movement training as a means of improving their mental and physical health and wellbeing. The Trust's other purpose was to maintain equal opportunities, health, safety and welfare of persons with learning disabilities involved in the YOU & ME system.

Initially the Trust set out to obtain funding to pilot the students' certificated programme. The idea was to accredit students who could demonstrate that they could achieve goals within their own range of abilities. In 1994 the Trust was granted European Social Fund (ESF) funding for 80 students and their trainers. This was carried out in collaboration with Cumbria Social Services and Westmorland Society for Mencap. The outcome was that 79 students, with moderate and severe learning difficulties, and profound and multiple disabilities, completed their OCNW Foundation Certificate with credits from the National Credit Framework (NCF).

This was one of the first ever Pre-Vocational Qualifications (PVQ) for such people. The PVQ programme and award with 2 NCF credits is intended to support, promote and enhance independent living skills for those with special needs and to aid progress towards vocational opportunities. The Whitehaven News commented: 'Students stepping up to receive certificates for work done on the YOU & ME project was the highlight of more than a years study and the first ever UK presentation under the scheme.' The look of pride on the faces of the candidates as they collected their certificates from the Manager of Cumbria Social Services Mrs. Maureen Maxey and the Co-ordinator of the Open College Mr. Jakes Makin was truly heart-warming. One could clearly see the handicaps many had overcome to demonstrate competence in the acquired skills. It was a real triumph for them and most rewarding for the trainers.

YOU & ME Students' Project

Karen Leslie, Senior Paediatric Physiotherapist, Lancaster, 1994/5 states:

'I have seen great improvements in the students' abilities in the following areas: balance, strength, coordination, body awareness, breath control, posture control, relaxation skills, and social skills. These abilities are necessary key skills to improve the students' vocational opportunities. Without doubt all these areas improve the students' quality of life.'

Kay Whittle, Director of Cumbria Social Services states:

'The YOU & ME system is the first such presentation that Cumbria Social Services have piloted in the UK, and it is now expected to be introduced for other people with learning disabilities throughout the country. I am pleased that so many people using our services have been able to gain a nationally recognised qualification.'

YOU & ME teaching is geared to: the development of personal and social skills; loosening-up the joints for assessment purposes and safety; the use of colour for relating the Postures to different parts of the body; practice of correct breathing; stillness and relaxation; involvement with selecting a sequence of Postures for Personal Whole-Body-Movement and finally performing the sequence. The YOU & ME colour-code recording system used for reviewing students' achievements clearly shows individual's progress through their regular practice. The course of training concludes with evaluating student's competence and areas of development, which is verified by an external moderator.

Experience has shown that persons with learning difficulties can gain great benefit from regular practice of the techniques, and that staff and parents can also benefit from teaching them, whether or not they have had any previous experience of yoga. They are of course particularly well qualified to teach the YOU & ME techniques to their charges because of the special relationship of understanding, closeness and trust that already exists.

The Trust was granted further ESF funding for piloting the Trainers' programme at OCNW Level 2 and Level 3. This certificated course was piloted in 1996–7 by myself with staff from Cumbria Social Services and volunteers from Westmorland Mencap Society. The six trainers were duly accredited competent YOU & ME Trainers and received their Trainers' certificates at Preliminary Level and Intermediate Level. Trainers' certificates were presented by top British comedy actor Harry Enfield.

Fortunately, I was given the freedom to operate the schemes by the Head of Training for Cumbria Social Services – Roger Dangerfield who had the vision for this programme to complement the existing services for the service users (i.e. clients with learning disabilities).

The following reports about these pilot-training projects were published in the Skill Journal – education, training and employment for people with learning difficulties and/or disabilities, Issue No. 61, June 1998, and FOCUS – a newsletter for staff working with people with visual and learning disabilities, February 1999, Number 26.

YOU & ME Trainers' Project

Six trainers gained through work experience the necessary knowledge and skills to teach the system with the utmost concern for the health, safety and welfare of their students, while gaining their own qualification.

Dr Janet Jones, OCNW, states:
'The programme for trainers is both comprehensive and effective. The trainers not only receive excellent instruction, but have to demonstrate and provide evidence of their aptitude and competence in the practical application of YOU & ME. The scheme has unquestionably expanded opportunities for both students and trainers.'

Maureen Maxey, Area Manager (North) Disability and Mental Health, Cumbria Social Services states:
'The YOU & ME Yoga project for trainers which took place during 1996 has enabled a member of Cumbria Social Services staff to obtain the Open College YOU & ME Level 3 qualification. This qualification has contributed to their obtaining Level 3 Day Service Officer qualification. The programme for trainers has been very successful not only for the students but also for the personal development of staff.'

Comments by some Trainers on the pilot-project
Elaine Harding, Community Nurse, Learning Disabilities Team, Whitehaven:
'The trainers' training on the YOU & ME course is of high quality, very intensive, informative and professional. The course covers every aspect of the teaching of YOU & ME to clients, highlighting the health, safety and welfare needs of clients. Attaining this knowledge enables the trainer to become competent and confident in teaching the course. This ensures the clients receive a high quality, safe-practice service from the trainers, allowing the clients to develop mentally, physically and socially at their own pace. This then enables the clients to become more independent in all areas of life skills.
'Many comments on this development have been observed and commented on by other professionals and carers. The YOU & ME Trainers' programme also contributed three Units towards my Level 3 'In Care' Nursing qualification.'

Janet Usher, Westmorland Society for Mencap:

'YOU & ME training is proving to be of great value to both the trainer and the client. It increases awareness of the clients' abilities by exploring the different parts of the body; and by the colour coding system, it enhances the clients' knowledge of his/her body and ways in which greater mobility can be achieved. The YOU & ME system is advantageous in teaching clients how to relax, and provides great fun with varied techniques to improve breathing. Relationships between client and trainer help to develop confidence and improve communication – thereby improving social skills. The system as a whole helps to improve quality of life. While I have been training as a trainer over the past fifteen months, I have seen a steady change and improvement in clients' ability and confidence.'

Nicola Watson, also from Westmorland Society for Mencap, continues:

'The YOU & ME programme of Whole-Body-Movement was introduced to a group of six club members in February 1996. Since then we have seen some remarkable changes among the class students as they progressed towards gaining their Foundation Level certificate.

'Reading through the record charts and reflecting on progress, it was satisfying to have given our students the opportunity to make improvements in many areas of their lives. Flexibility, coordination, balance and range of movement – all important for 'functional fitness' – have shown great improvement. Personal and social skills have developed as we have worked together as a group, and self-confidence, concentration and social interaction have been enhanced.

'D. reports that her backache is almost cured, and she is always smiling and laughing in the class. She allows physical help with the exercises, in contrast to much initial trepidation at any offer of help.

'D.W. shows a great improvement in her balance and control of movements. She is fiercely independent and always likes to try as many movements as she can. She now needs less support physically, and is generally stronger, so that she is better able to balance on her own.

'R. is now patient while others receive one-to-one help, and his behaviour is appropriate to what is going on throughout the session.

'A. knows where her diaphragm is and can now control it successfully when breathing and relaxing.

'G. is brighter and more confident, and is encouraged by the praise given to the range of movement he has achieved round his middle area. He tells us that tension in his shoulders is relieved by relaxation. He is more talkative and outgoing, having overcome his initial shyness. On leaving, he always comments how much he has enjoyed the session.'

The pilot-projects actually took a lot out of me. Being one of the first of its kind in the country, we were finding our way as we went. All the while under strict scrutiny from both OCNW, the accrediting body, and from the ESF – our funding body – who required everything to be recorded and accounted for. This was unexpected extra work that took up most of my spare time. Furthermore, payments from ESF took two-and-a-half years to come through from Brussels. This meant that I had to afford everything to keep the project running and I acquired a heavy overdraft to add to the struggle. However, through perseverance, the successful outcome of the two pilot training programmes made sense of it all in the end.

It was decided to wind-up the Trust because it had fulfilled its purpose in successfully piloting the training programmes for students and trainers.

Feedback from the Trainers of the pilot-project prompted me to complete the teaching materials for the training package to replace the loose-leaf handouts. I also endeavoured to reduce the record-keeping paperwork by designing an efficient system of recording charts, leaving more time for participants to enjoy their practice. Months turned into years whilst I worked at home completing this material.

At the time of writing, I am the only person qualified to teach the Trainers but it is not physically possible for me to provide the degree of support necessary during the training period to candidate trainers throughout the UK. I am now concentrating on developing a network of Tutors of Trainers qualified to carry on the YOU & ME training.

The Tutor of Trainers Programme

In October 1998 I submitted the Tutor of Trainers' Programme to OCNW in order to qualify YOU & ME Tutors in their prospective work places throughout the country. Due to the advanced nature of the Tutors training programme, this approval took nine months. There are several previously trained practitioners wanting to become qualified to teach YOU & ME to other staff members. To meet demand and provide the future professional Tutors of Trainers with underpinning knowledge of the YOU & ME Yoga system, the YOU & ME Advanced Certificated Programme for Tutor of Trainers was approved by OCNW in June 1999. This decision was recommended by various members of the Recognition and Access Panel, and two Directors and Founders of Yoga Institutions, a Training and Development Officer and a Physiotherapist.

In 1999 I won an Award from the Leadership Consortium, the Prince of Wales' Advisory Group on Disability for Leadership Development Training, which was sponsored by British Telecom (BT). This award introduced me to the value of communicating with a 'mentor', for one year, to help prioritise the activities in ones life. As part of the scheme I have had the privilege of being put in contact with various BT managerial experts to access appropriate information and advice. Consequently, the YOU & ME Trainers' and Tutor of Trainers' training programmes now includes coaching/assessment training days. These training days provide trainers with guidance, support and assessment of their abilities. When there are enough qualified Trainers, we also plan to provide trainee trainers with a Trainer – as their contact person for on-going support, and for dealing with any necessary advice when required.

YOU & ME Vocational Qualifications Update

The Trainers' programme enables trainers to gain recognition for their personal development, acquired skills and knowledge, and ability to teach the YOU & ME system to people with learning difficulties of varying ability. Once qualified, Trainers will be able to offer the Pre-Vocational – Foundation Level programme to their students.

The Tutor of Trainers Programme is to ensure YOU & ME Tutors have sufficient knowledge, understanding and skills, and qualities of leadership. Only qualified YOU & ME Trainers with considerable experience who wish to train others as YOU & ME Trainers will be approved to train in this Advanced Programme. Once qualified they will be able to offer the Preliminary and Intermediate Trainers' programmes.

Jakes Makin, as Director of Development states, June 1999:

The Open college of the North West has recognised and accredited the following programmes for the YOU & ME Trust:

1. Foundation Level for Students
2. Preliminary Level and Intermediate Level Trainer Programmes
3. Advanced Level Tutor Trainer Programme.

We consider these to be valuable programmes in supporting the learning of people with a range of developmental needs and abilities.

Summary of the System

The YOU & ME system of Whole-Body-Movement has been specially devised to meet the needs and develop the potential of persons with learning difficulties. It trains staff, carers and parents, together with their charges if desired, in a set of simple but effective techniques which have been carefully selected and arranged to relax, exercise and strengthen the whole of the body. Previous yoga experience is not necessary, just a commitment to learning, sharing and working with the students and others concerned. The YOU & ME system uses a combination of sound, colour and Whole-Body-Movement. Full details of the techniques are set out in the Trainer's Packs issued with the courses.

To sum up the advantages of YOU & ME: it is of personal benefit to all the participants, inexpensive to run and provides both trainers and students with nationally recognised qualifications with transferrable credits in Lifelong Learning.

Some Strategies for starting YOU & ME Yoga

The first step is to view the YOU & ME teaching video. The video – a valuable learning aid – constitutes a permanent record of the procedures and provides a means of learning the techniques. Note that it is a necessary prerequisite to study the video before attending the Trainers' programme.

Whether you wish to become fully qualified or not, it is advisable to practice the system's techniques – with reference to the Display Cards – for 20 minutes daily for at least three weeks following the training. Only then can a reasonably healthy person begin to feel the benefits of yoga and gain the confidence needed to start teaching YOU & ME Yoga to their charges. Yoga is such a fascinating subject which covers all aspects of our human potential. The practitioner does not need to undergo years of yoga training before they are able to pass on suitable techniques to their charges. However, it would be a good idea to attend a local yoga class – suitable for your level of ability – for personal development.

The Trainers' certificated programme involves the personal practise and study of YOU & ME Yoga and resulting in an in-depth understanding of the techniques – essential for teaching the system and for personal development and wellbeing.

When introducing YOU & ME to new students, trainers should try to work on a one-to-one basis. If this is not possible, trainers working on their own should aim to teach no more than three students. With one helper, trainers can teach six students – i.e. three extra per helper. Similarly, with two helpers, nine students can be taught. This will ensure that the abilities of students can be individually assessed and that health and safety rules can be strictly followed.

It is a good idea to acquire visual evidence of the student's performance from the outset – it rewards students to see their progress and is useful evidence for coursework and portfolios. Recording this evidence can be done photographically and by using the YOU & ME Colour-Code Recording System.

Amazing Grace in Meditation

It was Saturday, my first day off in ages, so I decided to lay in bed and watch my breathing and think about what I had been reading about in Howard Kent's book, *Breathe Better, Feel Better*. Howard mentions the all-pervading power of breathing and taking time to be still and quiet (meditating). He talks about making use of one's mental faculties to be steadfast in one's thinking and purpose in life, rather than focusing on the negative past and those things which cannot be changed. These things can be consciously released on the out-breath, wiping the slate clean – making space for welcoming in the new vital breath of wondrous life force. I had a dynamic experience of the breath and watching its direction; feeling the sensation of its movements and was totally immersed into it.

During this creative meditation I was taken in with my own self-awareness, found my own worth and life's purpose and felt grounded and well established. My YOU & ME Yoga Handbooks are complete and I am ready to share them with others. I experienced how well it was working with all concerned and the great interest, enthusiasm and appraisal.

I then felt the love for everyone using my system instead of the fear of anyone abusing my work. I had felt rather bruised and inhibited from previous experiences. Then in a moment I remembered how long it had been since I spent any time thinking about loving myself. For so long I had doubted and questioned myself. I was up against an unfair world because yoga for people with special needs does not fit into UK's statutory provision, in spite of my research, sixteen years ago, proving how effective it is in the Indian Special Needs curriculum! An overwhelming sense of love and gratefulness came to me, over and over again! I was past the moment of despair, with total awareness of the love and light of my existence. I was alive with so much to offer and share with love.

I shared my thoughts of love with all my family and friends; with my teachers and friends who have shared with me physically, mentally and spiritual, and especially those who have inspired me and reached my soul.

What a wonderful, liberating and powerful source our love for one another IS!

Further into this profound meditation session, my clarity of thought became so apparent that I could see into the future. I began to gain strength and hope to further my purpose and to see how to make it happen. It was my deepest desire to get my books published and to have a Yoga Centre for the third time. Unfortunately, a new Yoga Centre has not happened yet, so I have decided to hold local non/residential training courses and do itinerant teaching for a few months of the year, visiting appropriate individuals, venues and organisations where YOU & ME Yoga is required. With my PowerBook computer and the Internet, I am able to offer my services at home in the UK and abroad.

I am looking forward to the next phase of my life with the developments of the YOU & ME Yoga operational system. By establishing a professional YOU & ME Network of competent Trainers and Tutors, many more people will benefit from the practice. I welcome previously trained practitioners and newcomers to join this network to develop their practice of YOU & ME Yoga. I believe with competent and qualified Trainers and Tutors in this valuable field of work for disabled people, all my struggles developing the system will have been worth it!

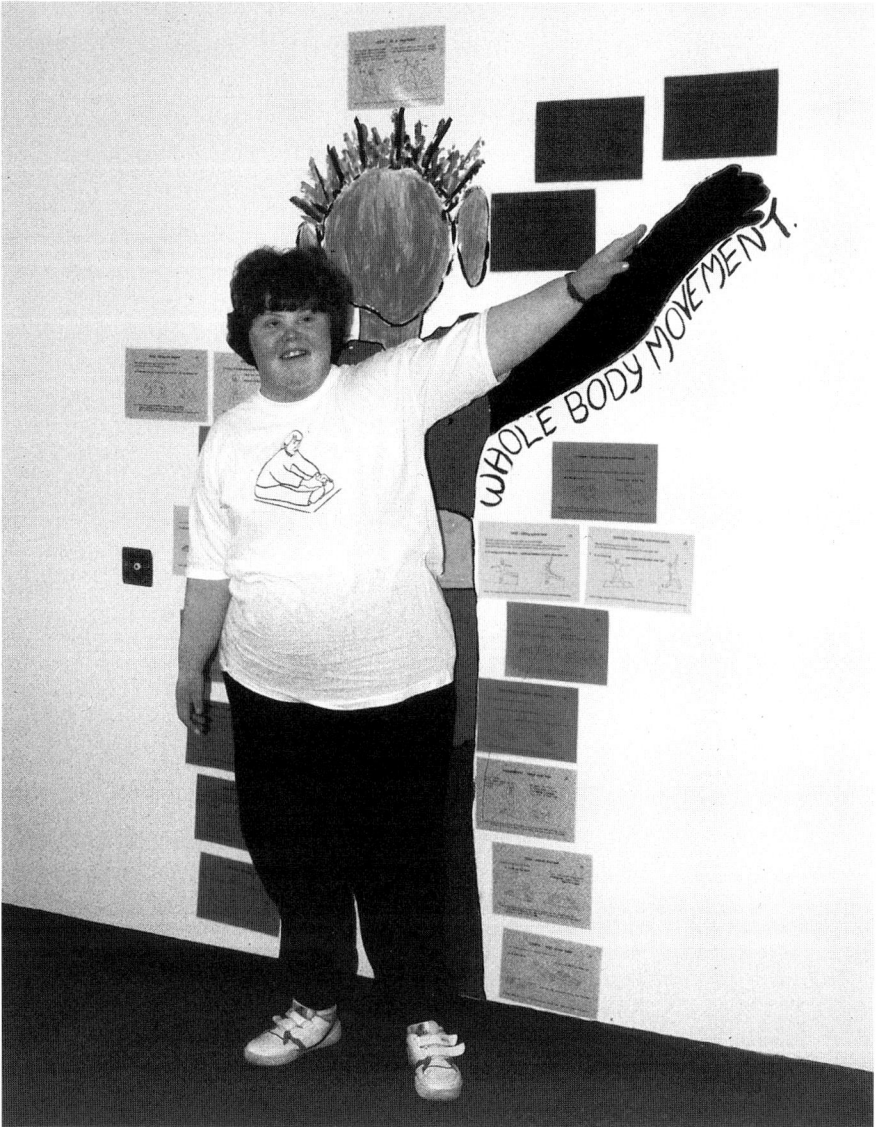

'Judith' on the front cover of the teaching video.

Part Five

Teaching Materials

CHAPTER TWENTY-TWO

Description of the YOU & ME Teaching Materials

The YOU & ME system and materials have been developed over several years. This development has involved study into yoga, special needs, disability, health, education, social welfare and information technology. Teaching and reference materials have been produced with the help and advice of many talented people.

YOU & ME Whole-Body-Movement Teaching Video

This 140-minute video, sponsored by Mencap City Foundation and assisted by LDHTV, features the YOU & ME Yoga system, using sound, colour and Whole-Body-Movement. It is designed for yoga practitioners, therapists, teachers, carers and parents of persons with learning difficulties and/or disabilities. The video shows people of all ages and abilities with conditions such as Down's Syndrome, autism, cerebral palsy, epilepsy, spasticity, paralysis; visual, aural and speech impairment and behavioural problems.

The video was recorded at special schools, adult training centres, residential homes and hospitals throughout the UK and Eire. Instruction is given by practitioners of the system using adaptations appropriate to their students and by some of the more advanced students themselves. Even those normally showing little response demonstrate how they are able to practise a thorough programme for the whole body. The techniques shown on the video help to bring about improved physical dexterity, coordination, and sensory awareness, and to make the students more calm, relaxed and confident.

The video consists of four parts:

- An introduction to the featured organisations;
- Preliminary movements for loosening up the joints, which are used for assessment;
- Twenty postures with adaptations necessary for various levels of ability and safety cautions;
- Methods of using the Colour-Code Instruction Pack for working out individual programmes of

Whole-Body-Movement.

N.B. There are 28 sections which can be studied and practised separately for experiential learning.

Flo Longhorn, Consultant in Special Education:

'The yoga video is superb, clear and concise, despite its length. I was particularly impressed with the use of special people giving some of the commentary. I also thought the way the participants exhibited their mastery of yoga, and delighted in their success, outstanding.

'This video is 'par excellence', a tribute to the YOU & ME system and sheer pleasure to watch.'

Loosener Display Cards – Instruction Pack

This pack contains a colour-code diagram to aid assessment of the student's ability and 22 A5 laminated double-sided coloured Display Cards. On one side the cards show clear illustrations of each stage of the movement, along with simple and precise instructions. The other side of the card lists the benefits that can accrue from the Loosener depending on the individual's abilities and amount of practice. The cards also detail guidelines for health and safety, and advice for students with specific disabilities from a physiotherapist.

Colour-Code Instruction Pack of the Postures

This pack contains a Colour-Code Guide booklet and 20 A5 laminated Display Cards illustrating the 20 Yoga Postures with simple, precise teaching instructions. These postures are used to create individual sequences of Whole-Body-Movement and suit the needs of students of all ages and levels of ability.

The booklet gives a choice of postures, indicates the order in which they should be performed and illustrates correct diaphragmatic breathing. The cards also detail physiological and psychological benefits and cautions as advised by the late Dr Frank Chandler, Medical Adviser of British Wheel of Yoga.

The protective lamination means that the cards can be displayed and used again and again.

Pat Pickering, Training Officer, Castleigh Day Centre, Nantwich:

'The Colour-Code Instruction Pack is essential for giving instructions for working out individual programme plans of Whole-Body-Movement. The pack explains everything very clearly, which enables trainers to select a suitable plan for people with learning difficulties or otherwise.'

YOU & ME Handbooks

The YOU & ME Handbooks will provide trainers with an invaluable resource for further reference and study. These books will enable therapists, trainers, carers, and parents to work together on the YOU & ME practices and are useful reference material for potential trainers who wish to become qualified in the YOU & ME system. These books are intended for practical application and reference, so that trainers, carers and parents (and the support/disciplinary team) can work on the YOU & ME practices, for the greater possible benefit to their charges.

The Handbooks comprise the complete works of the YOU & ME system and form competence-based yoga programmes. Note that only those that have successfully completed these courses will be able to describe their teaching method as the YOU & ME Yoga system. The trade name YOU & ME is a registered Trade Mark, and only when qualified under licence can it be used in any form what so ever.

My thanks go to Physiotherapist, Karen Leslie who provided the information on anatomy and physiology specified by Open College for health and safety. This information is presented in diagrammatic form along with guidelines for assessment of students abilities and for monitoring progress.

The training package contains over 4,000 illustrations showing how those of all ages and varying physical types manage to accomplish the techniques. The illustrations were taken from photographs of students practising their version of the techniques. Sanchia Lewis produced 800 of the drawings between 1985 and 1987. The remaining drawings were produced by Pauline Needham between 1988 and 2000.

The YOU & ME Training Handbooks comprise:

How to select sequences of Whole-Body-Movement
A reference book on how to devise individualised programme plans of the Postures using the Colour-Code Instruction Pack. Choice of Postures for Warming-Up and Winding-Down for each Main Posture are listed in order of preference. This is followed by the rationale for selection of each coloured Posture.

Learning Difficulties/Disabilities and Associated Conditions

Explanation of learning difficulties, *complete with case studies*, including: Down's syndrome, autism, cerebral palsy, and associated conditions such as epilepsy, challenging behaviour, deafness and visual disability.

Explanation of the Colour-Code

Use of colour. Colour and body awareness. Coloured movements. Colouring the different techniques and the bodily parts. Colouring and function of different coloured areas. Heaven on earth – our different states of being.

YOU & ME Recording Systems

A user-friendly comprehensive system for assessing the health, abilities, safety, welfare and progress of all students' yoga practice.

1. Using the recording system for the Looseners.

Assessment Guidelines for the Looseners – function of joints in relation to Looseners.

2. Using the Whole-Body-Movement recording system.

Assessment Guidelines for the Postures – function of joints in relation to Postures.

YOU & ME Whole-Body Looseners

Functions of the joints in relation to the Looseners. Cautions and conditions which affect the performance of the Looseners. Whole-Body Looseners explained. 1,500 line-drawing illustrations of people with learning disabilities, of all physical types, performing the Looseners or adaptations of them in their own special way.

YOU & ME Breathing and Relaxation Methods

Appropriate breathing and relaxation techniques. Facts about stress, and methods to cope with stress.

YOU & ME Yoga Postures

The appropriate yoga techniques suitable for people with learning difficulties. Whole-Body-Movement explained. Applied anatomy and the Postures – Muscles used when Performing the Twenty Postures. Cautions and conditions which affect performance of the Postures. 2,500 line-drawing illustrations of people with learning disabilities, of all physical types, performing the Postures or adaptations of them in their special way.

For further details contact www.youandmeyoga.com

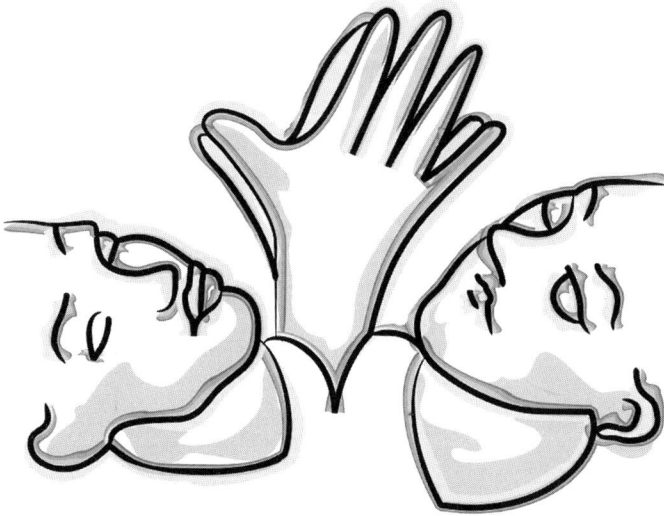

YOU&ME™

Yoga Opening Unfolding & Meaningful Experience

For current information on the training programmes and publications, please contact the YOU & ME Yoga web site address:

http://www.youandmeyoga.com